DESTINATION
Real Food:

Navigating Our Food System
and Restoring Soil to Improve Health

Angela Jenkins RD, LD

DEDICATION

This book is dedicated to my father and mother, Allan and Jane Ames who routinely provided the support and inspiration for me to become a lover of real food from a very young age. To my children, who have the opportunity to be part of the next generation of aware eaters. And to my "foodie" friends who inspire me weekly to continue to promote healthy, fun, food centric activities as well as opportunities to teach others. A specific shout out to my friends Paige, Jennifer, and Dawnnell, who provided some long hours of editing support; Jayma and Caroline for the venue to teach others about microbes in the soil and the connections between these microbes, soil, health, and the environment; Sarah, my perpetual garden buddy who is always up for the next soil adventure; and the early Well Fed Neighbor folks who started this journey with me from the beginning. I love you all dearly and appreciate you more than you know!

> "If we begin to nurture the behaviors that change our food experiences and food environments, we can facilitate lasting change, not just for us as individuals but for the greater good. Continuing to look at eating healthy just as a performance standard with possible long-term personal health outcomes, we'll inevitably fall short on the opportunities that have been laid before us as connected, social, environmentally concerned citizens." — Angela Jenkins

TABLE OF CONTENTS

1.
Journey Preparation.

Packing and Organizing

We all have an internal food narrative. That's to say, we all have a set of experiences, either imagined or real, throughout our lifetimes that drive our decision making around the food we put into our bodies. Think back to your first food memory. Was it associated with some sort of fun time or nostalgic tradition your family had? Or remember the first time you had an ice cream sundae slathered with all the thick chocolate fudge topping, nuts, and a cherry on top. That slight stomach ache became a nostalgic memory because one never knew when the next one would be offered. There didn't used to be fast-food restaurants serving ice cream on every other corner. Now, think back to the first time you were offered a food that tasted awful to you. How long was it before you tried that food again? Perhaps it was given to you before your taste buds were fully developed and, therefore, you couldn't fully appreciate the complexity of flavor it had to offer. Now, it's no longer something that you would be willing to try again years later.

These are the experiences that continue to influence our food choices today.

Think back again now to how your family managed food in your house. Did your family eat breakfast every day or was this something that wasn't emphasized as important? Did your parents always buy that next trendy food product on the market? Did your family have a garden? Were you allowed to be a part of the planting and harvesting of food from that garden? If so, was this something that you enjoyed or didn't enjoy? Many times, our enjoyment around food is dictated by some distant memory of how the family you grew up in approached food. If gardening was a fun, engaging event at your house, you would be more likely to carry it into adulthood, as opposed to the family that treated it as something that was just a chore and had to be managed. Was there any emphasis placed on nutritious food at all in your house growing up, or was someone always on a diet? Did your family eat together consistently? Was it fun or was it stressful?

In some families, gathering and eating together was the time that some major family decisions were made, and this time was quite protected regarding attendance. Yet other families have policies around not getting dessert unless everything was eaten on your plate, otherwise known as "the clean plate club." One of my personal favorites is the Irish potato famine shaming into eating all the potatoes on your plate. Perhaps, had we lived through these times, a greater appreciation of the potato could be offered back in the form of always finishing the potatoes on your plate?

These are the sorts of experiences that initially shape our conversation and action around how to manage food in our lives. This internal food narrative can be conscious or subconscious. Many times, if we're unconsciously making these decisions, then food tends to be unimportant, just filling hungry stomachs, unless you were fortunate to grow up in a food environment where healthy food was always in the forefront of the conversation. Statistically, however, this isn't likely to be the case. Our lives have become so busy, less "food-centric," which makes the sit-at-home meal with the entire family somewhat of a thing of the past. We run through fast-food lines with phones in hand looking up the next stop or a response to some social media post, inching forward to receive a bag through a window. Eating in the seat of a vehicle is more the norm, squeezing in one more stop before heading home late at night.

Just as every person has an internal narrative around food, every family has food roots separate from how we were raised. That is, every family has some history with food and food production. Every family has to have food roots because this was the only way food existed just 3-4 generations back. How has this shaped your understanding and belief systems around food? Most commonly, the generational rural farm has long since been sold for a mighty profit because of the incremental creeping in of the concrete jungle or urban sprawl known as urban development or "progress." Cities become larger and farming land in operation diminishes. Farming is long hours or heavy labor, intensive work, for an offer of little bottom line apparent financial gain. Some folks still live on a farm but no longer have it in agricultural production because of that same hard work. Those who have maintained production on a large scale often have succumbed to the larger agricultural narrative that consistent amendments are needed at large cost. This is just how it's always been, so this is just how it's done. Least commonly, farmers have hung in there plugging away, seeing it as the only way to fight back to ensure real food is available desiring to be a part of the agricultural, environmental, community, and health solution for the planet. This latter scenario needs to become the most common rather than the least, which I will write a lot about in the coming pages.

Meanwhile and gradually over the last 70 years, shelves at the grocery stores are being filled with new and trendy products, enticingly packaged to allure the shopper unaware that the nutritional value of the food on those shelves has deteriorated dramatically. This creeping in of low-quality foods in high volume has occurred through a series of policy changes on national, state, and community levels, but we've been too busy to notice.

Often, food labels tell a story about the product that's more designed to pull at your heart strings rather than educate about the food actually grown or how it was processed. An educated decision surrounding healthy food choices isn't really possible in America as we have legislated that opportunity away. We often hear of our soils being depleted, but are they? And what can an average consumer do about this if anything? Shouldn't our internal narrative encourage us to know where our food is coming from and what's happening to it prior to placement on a grocery store shelf? Begin thinking about your story and where you're in this continuum known as your internal food narrative and food roots. I'll tell you a bit about mine.

My Food Narrative

I still have a picture of my great grandfather and me when I was 10 years old on a beach in Jonesport, Maine. He was sitting in an Adirondack chair smiling, wearing his ball cap. I'm awkwardly posed next to him but also smiling with my teeth seemingly too big for my head wearing a large-collared shirt trendy for the 70's. Our family had decided it was a good idea to gather for a reunion in the place that our family remembers it was from. It was also likely that it was the only way to ensure that older members of the family were able to be in attendance. I remember very little of the experience at the reunion, but the picture was endearing because my great grandfather was 107 years old.

My great grandfather, Grover Cleveland Higgins or "Cleve" was a lobsterman, a farmer, and a gardener. He got up at the crack of dawn and was out on the lobster boats, setting up or picking up lobster traps in whatever weather necessary to keep a roof over his family's head. He worked all morning and then off the boats and back for lunch. I remember stories about him when we were sitting around "camp," the family cottage in Maine. He would take a shot of whiskey and a nap every day around noon and then head out to the fields to work. He actually made his own lobster traps in the barn out of bent spruce harvested on the property and weaved the netting with carefully placed bowline knots to create these traps that were the foundation of his livelihood. Every few days, he would place the traps, then harvest them and bring them to a local market and do it over again the next day.

Georgia, Cleve's forever bride, would bake bread from scratch daily. Other local foods that they didn't produce out of their own garden were traded or bartered for other items that were needed. They also raised pigs, cattle, and sheep on the farm. This is how they spent their day, in nonstop planning centered around food production, harvesting, or planning food for the future. Today, this would be known as subsistence living or homesteading. Much of rural America functioned this way.

In the 1940s, almost everyone had a farm or a garden of some sort because industrialized food was really just on the verge of becoming a booming business. They had to garden. There were no convenience stores for one-stop shopping to grab a breakfast burrito, fill up the gas tank, and head to work. Small, medium, and large farms existed all along the Maine coastline. People worked hard outside day in and day out, cultivating what they could on the land that they had because there was no grand back up plan. Maine soil is notoriously rocky but also acidic and tough to grow food in, but its most famous crop appreciates this kind of soil: the Maine blueberry. Left behind by the glaciers hundreds of thousands of years ago, they've now become a major cash crop for the state.

I remember as a child and actually well into my adult years, paddling across the lake from camp to "Blueberry Island" where we would pick blueberries until we had buckets full. We would then paddle back to camp and make the most delicious blueberry pies. They were most delicious because not only had we worked hard personally to pick them but there's nothing like a blueberry pie made from Maine blueberries. Maine blueberries are smaller, more nutritious, and more delicious than larger blueberry varieties. To this day, if we're in Maine, during picking season, which runs from the third week in July through early September, we pick berries on the island.

Jonesport, Maine, was a major fishing port back at the turn of the 20th century, but even by the time my picture with Grover Cleveland was taken in the late 1970s, the town was in major decline. Larger, more accessible ports along the coast of Maine began to become available and the family business of lobstering became less necessary from that particular location. People began to move away, toward the larger cities where they could make more money, working for someone else in fewer hours per day. The number of farms began to decline and continues to decline to this day. The *2017 Census of Agriculture Profile*[1] report shows a 22% decline in the number of acres being farmed from 2007-2017 in Washington County where Jonesport resides. Today the city also has limited

---

[1] USDA ERS Atlas. https://www.nass.usda.gov/Publications/AgCensus/2017/Online_Resources/County_Profiles/index.php

access to grocery stores and is considered a food desert, meaning that most folks don't live within 10 miles of a grocery store. This story is a familiar one across the country all over rural America.

My great grandfather never left Jonesport for this exodus in search of better opportunity but my grandparents after they married did and moved 80 miles west to Brewer, Maine. Here, they raised three children, including my father, who was the eldest. My father, in turn, moved with my mother down to Reading, Massachusetts, where I spent my entire childhood in the same house at 14 Arnold Avenue. I was the middle child in a very middle-class upbringing in suburban America. My mother was a stay-at-home mother until we attended high school and then she started working because we were never home anymore.

While we departed from our roots in Jonesport, there was always this ongoing conversation or action around food in our house. Every year, my parents planted an extremely large garden. I remember the incredible bounty that came from that 30-30-foot plot on the side of the house. There were always marigolds planted around the perimeter of the garden, which I now understand help to attract bees and protect the tomatoes from invading nematodes. This is known as companion planting whereby different plants have a symbiotic relationship with one another. There were always tomatoes, peppers, cucumbers, and greens of some sort, usually Swiss chard. As a child, I remember being asked to pick foods from the garden and bring them to my mother so dinner could be prepared. When I was younger, my mother did all the cooking and only on a rare occasion do I remember ever eating outside of our home until we were well into high school.

My father also enjoyed cooking occasionally when he was home, engineering and naming his own dishes such as WIGLOPS which was an acronym for every ingredient in the recipe. The W stood for wine, which made it a purple noodle dish filled with peas and onions necessitating a hearty, perhaps smirky, discussion over what else this dish contained at the dinner table. My mother canned tomatoes for spaghetti sauce that we ate year-round, and she made applesauce from the large apple tree in the backyard. I loved this applesauce. I would have eaten it by the gallons except for the natural side effects of eating too much. Periodically, we would have Super Sandwich night too. This was an opportunity for us to concoct our own sandwich from whatever deli meats my mother purchased for this event as well as specialty toppings and extra vegetables to pile high on these sandwiches. Quite often, I was unable to fit my mouth around the sandwich, and many of the toppings that spilled out had to be eaten separate from the sandwich itself, usually with my fingers.

This was the food environment that I grew up in. We didn't necessarily know who produced all of our food, but we certainly made family efforts to capitalize on the resources that were available to us at the time. While the culture around us at 14 Arnold Avenue was changing somewhat toward a society of convenience, we weren't that unusual. It was still less expensive to grow much of our own food, and we knew how. These are just snippets from my personal food journey shared with the intention of encouraging others to think about their own experiences that formed their relationship with food. Reflecting on the connections in and around food choices and why we choose what we choose is helpful in understanding our own behaviors and how we got where we are in our own health situations.

All Health Is Local

Food environments are important because they're the most immediate influence on our health. Whether it's home, school, the office, cafeteria, or the local grocery store, this access to food dictates much of what we eat. In the home I grew up in, there was always plenty of healthy, nutritious food available in our home. We brought our lunches to school, and, although we bought quite a bit of food from the grocery store even with the garden in the backyard, my parents always emphasized healthy food options, and this is what made it back into the house. We ate and tried new dishes throughout the month, and we ate together almost every evening. Most everything we ate was made from scratch, except for bread and any desserts if there were such an occasion. This is not even close to the situation in America today.

There has been a significant and nutritionally detrimental departure from how we used to eat in America. A 2017 report from the USDA Economic Research Service indicated that we now spend 54% of our food dollars outside the home in restaurants.[2] This means that we're essentially not in charge of most of what's being put in our bodies. Assuming that we all have access to the food we want, it's not that we aren't making conscious decisions about what to eat, but more that it's not possible to be aware of what we're eating because we're eating outside of our homes. Many times, people don't have access to the foods they want. In this case, the nutritional quality of what's available is perhaps even worse. In the 1940s, we ate approximately half this amount outside the home. This one statistic really explains a lot. As a practicing dietitian for 30 years, I've watched fad diets, food trends, and all sorts of hocus pocus around food and dieting come and go. Meanwhile, the foundation of our healthy food behaviors that keep us engaged with food and wanting to take care of ourselves holistically has degraded gradually over time. We eat out too much and it's affecting our health negatively and substantially.

To add a layer of concern, there have been changes around how our foods are grown and raised. A tomato in the 1940s or in my parents' garden growing up isn't the same as a tomato today from the grocery store. So how do we know how to choose a tomato? Looks like a tomato, smells like a tomato, kind of tastes like a tomato, must be a tomato, right? Unless you're buying organic, the tomato that you're eating is most likely genetically modified or a hybrid, grown in depleted soil with pesticides and shipped halfway across the country in ethylene gas. Is this tomato as healthy a choice as a tomato grown locally and regeneratively or organically? The answer is no. It doesn't have the same nutritional content as a tomato grown in your own backyard, picked at the peak of ripeness. And, the

---

[2] New US Food Expenditure Estimates Find Food Away From Home Spending Higher Than Previous Estimates, by Howard Elitzak and Abigail Okrent, USDA, ERS, November 5, 2018. https://www.ers.usda.gov/amber-waves/2018/november/new-us-food-expenditure-estimates-find-food-away-from-home-spending-is-higher-than-previous-estimates/

pesticide residues on it have the potential to disrupt your microbiome (beneficial gut bacteria) as well as your endocrine system.

Another example would be that the T-bone steak from your favorite restaurant isn't the same as a T-bone steak from an organic grass-fed beef producer at the farmer's market down the road. Those ever-important Omega-3 fatty acids are higher in the grass-fed T-bone steaks. T-bone steaks are no easier to choose than those tomatoes. When you're standing at the meat counter trying to figure out which steak to choose and none of them are labeled, how do you know what to ask? And when you do, will the butcher know the answer? My experience is that most of the time, they don't. So, what's a consumer to do who wants to improve health by making wiser food decisions? Many times, people choose the cheapest option because this information is not available, not recognizing that the ultimate cost is that of their health later on down the line. Knowing that how we grow our food and raise our food affects our health dramatically only goes as far as the questions that can be answered to guide our food choices. As Ann Wigmore from the Natural Health Institute once said, "The food you eat can be either the safest and most powerful form of medicine or the slowest form of poison." If given a choice, which would you choose?

Our modern-day food system favors single bottom line agricultural food production, which means high profit margins with little consideration for anything else. Efficiency is most important, which leaves any health or environmental concern associated with food production or equity by the wayside. This goes on essentially unnoticed because we Americans aren't in charge of our food anymore. We have, for all intents and purposes, outsourced our food and our health to other people to manage. This outsourcing is taking its toll because it looks like a tomato or a T-bone steak but how it was grown and raised much of the time isn't conducive to supporting not only our health but also the health of the planet. One would think that, with all the modern agricultural and medical technology available to us, we would be the healthiest country on the planet, but we're not even close; we're 45th. The issue is likely multifactorial in nature, and I'll attempt to unfold some of it in the coming pages.

The choices that we're making by supporting these agricultural systems are degrading not only our health but our environment as well. The GREEN REVOLUTION whereby industrialized agriculture began adding inorganic amendments to the soil rather than replacing the biology and organic matter in the soil has perpetuated further decline in not only our soil base but also our air and water quality. How you or your neighbor treats their land directly impacts your health, but, often, we don't equate the two. This outsourcing or industrialization of our food in America has left us separated from understanding what influences food production, how it's produced, its availability within close proximity, and even how to choose well for ourselves and support community endeavors or the environment.

With this in mind, eating food has become somewhat of a political act. Where we spend our food dollars reinforces the support for that food system. It's really that simple. If we buy a lot of processed food, we support the industrialized and highly mechanized food system. If we buy local, regenerative foods, we support local food systems. We support our neighbors. We support our people. The American consumer is the largest economic engine on the planet. And if we decide as consumers to support local, regeneratively raised food, the market will have no choice but to respond. We, unfortunately, get wrapped up in the new, trendy food items on the market that have diminished food values because they're cool rather than nutritious. And we outsource our health because of it.

Our conventional medical care has also been outsourced. One of my great concerns as a dietitian for 30 years is the almost complete lack of trust from physicians that food is, in fact, medicine. Would it surprise you to know that most physicians aren't trained in nutrition? Some may have one class, and, because of this lack of education, if someone has a heart disease, medication is prescribed. If someone has gastroesophageal reflux, medication is prescribed. If someone has high blood pressure, medication is prescribed. In each of these cases, these people should have been prescribed a new lifestyle and provided some tools for success or, at least, a referral to someone who could help evaluate lifestyle changes, but, in most cases, it's never mentioned. Perhaps it's just easier to pop a pill, but the resulting situation is, unfortunately, that Americans are living longer than ever before, but they're sicker than ever before and taking more medication than ever before. The next generation isn't expected to live longer than the current generation. How can this be happening in the land of plenty where we have access to the best medical care and an abundant food supply?

Most of my career I spent in inpatient clinical settings in a large medical institution in SW Missouri where I specialized in pediatrics for 16 years and allocated quite a bit of time to research why we were experiencing some of the greatest increases in obesity in our children in America. Something didn't add up. These kids weren't eating that much. Other factors had to be at play. Meanwhile, I kept researching and asking questions about our food supply, which led down the path of understanding that our industrialized food system is compromising not only our health but also our environment, communities, and local farms. The intricate webs of our food system are sometimes hard to define, unless we immerse ourselves within the inner workings of the system itself.

For this reason, in 2013, I facilitated the start-up of the Ozarks Regional Food Policy Council (ORFPC) that brought together 50 organizations in the SW Missouri region to accomplish the first food system assessment in our area to help define the health needs of our community relative to our local food system. This was where we, as a community, defined what we saw as a viable solution to improving the health of our children. The small, vibrant, regenerative farm was central for the creation of food that was healthy and available to the community. This is the same concept from Jonesport Maine or any other rural community where people supported one another and produced high-quality food. This concept made more sense to support the health of our children, in particular, those most vulnerable to eating the poor quality food that's more widely available.

The local food system assessment gave our community some actionable direction on how to support the health of our children and our people. This issue with our health and local food systems has much to offer the health of our children here in SW Missouri and also every community around the nation. You see, all health is local. While the industrialized food system is far reaching and impacts our health due to wide scale availability, the greatest impacts are those that are right around us in our immediate vicinity.

Bringing Health Home

The blueberry farmers in Maine ultimately found a way to make harvesting those small delicious, incredibly nutritious nuggets more efficient. I suspect that, had there been an easier way to be a lobsterman and work the farm, my great grandfather would have chosen this path. This was hard, back-breaking work without the farm equipment that we now have available to us today. Growing a garden on the coast of Maine is meticulous and consistently amenable at best. But what if this garden and his hard work translated into his health and longevity? What if the garden at our house in Reading was literally shaping our health outcomes because of the lifestyle our parents and grandparents led before us?

Studies have proven that gardening contributes to our health outcomes. A 2017 meta-analysis[3] reported a wide range of health outcomes, such as reductions in depression, anxiety, and body mass index as well as increases in life satisfaction, quality of life, and sense of community associated with gardening. Studies have shown that this impact is directly related to the microbiome of the soil and perhaps why so many people garden to relieve stress and leave their gloves off when gardening. Thankfully, statistics show that, on the whole, there has been an increase in the number of backyard gardens, but it still only translates to one out of three people. This means that there are over 200 million people not putting their hands in the soil or connecting with food in this capacity or what I call building a relationship with real food. Not everyone will be able to have a backyard garden, but there are other options that will be brought to light through these pages.

_____

[3] Masashi S, Gaston, K. J., & Yamaura, Y. Gardening Is Beneficial for Health: A Meta-Analysis, *Preventive Medicine Reports*, Volume 5, 2017, Pages 92-99. https://www.sciencedirect.com/science/article/pii/S2211335516301401

Just as all health is local, everyone has a food journey. Everyone's journey will be different on an interpersonal level, but the overarching external influences are essentially the same. In America, we have national food policies that impact not only what's grown but also how it's grown. Then, within each state, how agriculture is approached has a separate set of policies, and, then again, within each community, there are another subset of influences. The ultimate choice, however, is yours regarding what you bring into your home, your food environment, as well as how you prepare it. Therefore, choose a food environment that connects with family at a sit-down meal or in the yard, conversing over the events or stressors of the day, being champions for one another, and with foods that are raised regeneratively, connecting farm and family as well as community local food economic endeavors.

Pockets of communities and cities are connecting in this capacity around the country by trying to build regional food systems. As you progress through these pages, you will find stories of local successes in SW Missouri as well as failures, but perhaps the most important takeaway should be that the reconnection with our food and who produces it is fundamental to the recovery of our health, our communities, and our ecosystems. The paradigm shifts toward eating with a purpose; the purpose of supporting the regional food system, rebuilding the soil rather than trying to grow in dirt and expecting our food to be healthy and nutritious.

Even though my life's work has been as a dietitian, this isn't the average book about food. I would prefer to look at it as a navigational tool for you to choose your direction through our food system to decide how to influence your own health, community, and the environment with food choices. This book is for people who want to know where their health got lost in an industrialized food system and a drug-obsessed medical care system so they can regain it and keep it from happening again. Making more mindful, conscious "food-centric" life choices also supports the food systems that produce real food that, in turn, nurtures rather than degrades health and the environment. It's for people who want a foundational, actionable lifestyle plan that helps to redefine what keeps us eating what we should eat and connecting with our community. Eating well is one of the most fundamental supports of life, but, in America, our stomachs are full but our health is failing. Becoming more connected with where our food is coming from and how it's raised and produced can improve our health greatly, especially if done with community and the environment in mind.

2.
You Can't Get There From Here....GPS Is Broken

You can't get there from here. I always loved it when someone said that to me. In my pragmatic mind, any place is accessible with the right mode of transportation, a determined spirit and plenty of time. Let's imagine that there's an island off the coast of Maine named Vitality. Vitality is this beautiful place with large pine trees but also plenty of open fields. In these fields is an abundance of fresh fruit trees, blueberries perhaps, and vegetables with farm animals roaming around grazing on whatever they would normally like to eat like grass and acorns. The sweet smell of bread baking is waffling through the air as you walk closer to one of the shops downtown. The local coffee shop has made the best bread and the best coffee for decades, and folks gather to cuss and discuss what happened at the community picnic the day before.

Every person here contributes in some way to the food system or community on the island. Several people have their own greenhouse operations for four-season vegetable production, several are fishermen, some keep bees in addition to their other daily work endeavors, several bake their own bread not only for personal consumption but also for commercial sale to the local grocery store or cooperative, and yet another owns a processing plant to process all the local meats that are raised. Agricultural inputs come from other community members such as wood chips from the local tree service or manure from the local dairy or chicken farm. The food system is set up to cycle money back to the community supporting one another rather than going to a big box store. In this way, the food system helps to build community because everyone knows that their business will be supported rather than outsourced. This is a place where its citizens frequently eat together, work hard, but also support one another through the trials that life has to offer. It's going to be some work to get to the island, but it's worth the time and effort. Nobody goes hungry here, despite there being no subsidies from the federal government to grow food.

In the agrarian-based community, every community member provides value but is also valued. The mailman lives in the community and knows everyone by name. While people still gossip in Vitality, they all know that, at the end of the day, the community around them supports their effort and endeavors because they all choose to be in this environment. Sounds a little like Mayberry, doesn't it? To be clear, and to differentiate from a commune, this place of Vitality is full of legitimate businesses that purposefully support one another with needed products and services within a local or regional operating radius. This used to be how rural America thrived for a century or so. Why would this place be appealing? Vitality supports the health of the community, the economy, the environment and its people. Here these communities cultivate not only food but trust.

Places somewhat like this are popping up all around the country under a variety of different names, such as agriburbia or agrihoods, teeming with people who raise food regeneratively and couple it with land development practices that help to build purposeful communities. We Americans love our gated communities around golf courses. Why not develop purposefully around agricultural operations? Regenerative agriculture is different even from organic agriculture, as it actively seeks to support soil health and diversity, healthy ecosystems, and water quality, which, in turn, aids in the production of a higher nutritional value food product. Regenerative means just that. Regeneration of the soil and the systems that support it. This will be defined more extensively in coming chapters.

Now, in order to get to Vitality, you've been provided with a GPS unit that has been disabled and keeps sending you to the front door of a Walmart Supercenter. You can see the ferry going off in the distance to the island of Vitality, but you just can't make it to the boat ramp. What's the likelihood you're going to make it to Vitality? Most of us aren't likely to make it to the island because our largest supported food system in America doesn't support our health, and, in many cases, people are totally unaware.

An easy way to remember what a food system is to think of it as the path that a food travels from its conception till it enters your stomach. Some buzz terms frequently used are Farm to Table, Farm to School, Farm to Fork, Farm to Fridge, Dirt to Door, or Ground to Grub. A food system explains what happens to your food from the moment it's conceived or sprouted to the time it's presented on the table. This includes growing, harvesting, processing, packaging, transporting, marketing, consuming, and disposing or composting of food. So, our food travels from the ground and then, depending upon what its destiny is, ends up eventually back in the ground in some form. In order to accomplish an industrialized food system, there must be large-scale, wide-reaching food chains set up that allow for the distribution of these food products. Food supply chains are the processes set up to get food after it's grown and harvested to the processor, then from the processor to the grocery store for the consumer to purchase. Different foods will have different food supply chains, as foods are raised and grown differently, but, for the most part, the inputs into these systems are just from large-scale conventional, industrialized agriculture. To put it simply, this system cannot be bothered with the small diversified regenerative farm operation that I continually promote in this book as the essential steps forward to nurture health and the environment.

Perhaps it sounds strange that our food system is broken when there are so many "food-like substances" on the shelves of the grocery store. The brokenness of this system was never more evident than during the COVID-19 crisis; so, Chapter 5 was added to this book to illustrate this. The question remains, however, does this system provide real food? Remember the tomato and the T-bone? Food by definition should nourish our bodies, but we, as a nation, aren't well and the food system currently in operation is a major contributor to the problem. We're overfed but undernourished. Let's take a look at the national food policy that dictates what's grown in this country and then gradually distill it down to how food is managed in our homes to uncover a bit more of what's keeping us from Vitality.

Federal Policy

When thinking of the word "policy," most generally think of something that's restrictive. My place of work, at one point, had a policy that women couldn't wear skirts above the knee. All skirts had to be below the knee, or it was suggested that you should go home and change. Policy certainly can be restrictive, but it can also be defined in ways that encourage growth and development. Initially, the examples provided in the first several chapters will discuss some of these more restrictive policies, but I will also provide examples of how policy can be used to facilitate economic and community growth later in this book.

Our federal food policy is essentially the Global Positioning System (GPS) on our journey to Vitality. Our GPS directs mass production of crops in the United States as is defined by the Farm Bill. The Farm Bill that's renewed every four years dictates what crops or foods are grown in our country via subsidies as well as what supplemental nutrition assistance programs are supported and to what degree. The latest Farm Bill renewed on December 18, 2018, was renewed for what's projected to cost $867 billion over the next 10 years.[4] The first ever Farm Bill was initiated in 1933 in an effort to support struggling farmers through the dust bowl days and the great depression of 1929. The bill ensured that farmers were supported in their food production and there was food consistently available to US citizens but not an abundance of any one crop. This is also where the understanding became widely accepted that having an abundance of a crop actually forces the price of a crop down. Some farmers were incentivized to produce less or not at all and still got paid.

The lion's share of the Farm Bill is now supplemental assistance programs such as SNAP otherwise known as food stamps, and programs such as Women, Infants and Children or WIC. A whopping $664 Billion goes to nutrition programs. We'll talk about this a little more in the coming pages. The Farm Bill

---

[4] National Sustainable Agriculture Coalition Blog, National Farm Bill by Numbers, December 2018.http://sustainableagriculture.net/blog/2018-farm-bill-by-the-numbers/

also has provisions for commodity programs, crop insurance, and conservation programs. Commodities received $64.6 billion, crop Insurance $77.9 billion and conservation programs $59.6 billion. Let's whittle this down a little bit further.

Commodity programs provide subsidies for what's grown in America. The crops that are subsidized in order from greatest to least allocation of funds are: corn, wheat, soy, rice, livestock, sorghum, dairy, peanuts, barley, sunflower, canola, oats and apples. Every state will have a different greatest to least allocation relative to what is grown in each state. Who is receiving these subsidies might interest you. Many of the same farmers receive subsidies year after year with the top 20 allocations between $5-16 million over the 18 years.[5] Some of these farms are owned by millionaires and billionaires. The money provided to these farmers isn't distributed based on greatest need or how the crop is grown, conventional vs. regeneratively vs. organic, or whether previous subsidies have been received and how much.

Why does all this matter to our health? We eat what we subsidize in America, and the largest supported food system doesn't support healthy food options.[6] And to be clear, subsidization of any system creates some enormous imbalances within sectors that are subsidized depending directly upon how that subsidization is managed. We have large amounts of processed food made from these subsidized crops, such as corn, wheat, and soy, as well as highly processed oils, such as canola and sunflower oils, and what I call industrialized meat and dairy products. Because they're subsidized, foods made from these ingredients are widely available at a lower cost than unsubsidized foods. Many times, when I'm

---

[5] Mapping the US Subsidy $1 Milion Club, *Forbes*, Adam Andrezejewski, August 14, 2018. https://www.forbes.com/sites/adamandrzejewski/2018/08/14/mapping-the-u-s-farm-subsidy-1-million-club/#1224715b3efc

[6] Do, W. L., Bullard, K. M., Stein, A. D., Ali, M. K., Narayan, K. M. V., & Siegel, K. R. Consumption of Foods Derived from Subsidized Crops Remains Associated with Cardiometabolic Risk: An Update on the Evidence Using the National Health and Nutrition Examination Survey 2009-2014. *Nutrients*. 2020 Oct 23; 12(11): 3244. https://www.ncbi.nlm.nih.gov/pmc/articles/PMC7690710/

consulting with my patients, I recommend that they remove these food products from their diet because they can cause problems with their health. I'll explain more about why from a health standpoint in the coming chapters.

The people who gain the most from our current national food system are large farms that produce one food product, otherwise known as a monocrop. This is because the small- to medium-sized diversified farm cannot capitalize on this system even remotely close to how large agriculture or industrial agribusiness can. Not only do monocrops farms not support the health of the soil but they can actually cause disruptions within our ecosystems as well as producing nutritionally inferior food products depending upon how the farms are managed. The current Farm Bill supports farmers who produce crops that "can be insured," which discourages diversity. Forty percent of our on-farm biology has been wiped out in 50 years. It's not that a diversified farm couldn't be insured but that it becomes complicated relative to the different crops and their losses and is accomplished with fixed pricing; therefore, it's generally not approached by the larger system. Diversity supports the ecosystem as well as the offering of multiple product lines that support diversity in the diet as well.

All isn't lost, however. Local and regional food systems that would support the smaller diversified farm were introduced in 2009 to the Farm Bill 76 years later. Better late than never I always say. The 2018 Farm Bill provided permanent funding to help support smaller non-diversified producers as well. These programs are covered mainly under conservation, depending on how one splits it up, representing approximately $2.55 billion. For perspective, in the next 10 years, that doesn't even amount to 0.33% of the total Farm Bill. Sadly, those who have watched this funding for decades would call this progress in the right direction because it's an improvement over what we had previously available to those interested in having sustainability supported.

So, from the food system standpoint, where does all this food that's produced from monocrops go from the field? What's their food chain? Different crops go to different places but, for example, let's follow corn from field to, well, sometimes fork. I say sometimes because the largest percentage of corn is never actually eaten by us. It's important to understand that with corn, like many other subsidized foods, a large percentage are genetically modified organisms or GMO and don't support diversity. It's harvested from the field and goes to one of three places: our tables, our gas tanks, or feed for animals. It's challenging to determine how much of what goes where from the data provided from the USDA Economic Research Service (ERS), but in 2018, 33% of corn production went to biofuel, 33% as animal feed, and then 33% to our tables in the form of highly processed foods, such as high fructose corn syrup and cereals, or to seed or even exports.[7]

According to the USDA ERS, it's the most widely produced grain in America, accounting for 95% of grain produced in our country. It's interesting to note that America also imported approximately 874 to 1,000 metric tons of corn in 2018 despite our mass production of corn that isn't eaten. I emailed the ERS about why we would need to import any corn and they indicated that much of this is organic corn. One might wonder why we would need to import organic corn. It's certainly not that we aren't capable of producing organic corn but perhaps more that we just don't produce it. I emailed ERS about this as well but received no response. So, this will leave us guessing about the reasons for this, but I suspect the coming paragraphs may explain some of the cause. Our food system isn't well organized at very least and certainly not organized to support health. We have continually given up more and more land every year since the early 1990's to provide more space for producing corn, diminishing other grain crops never landing on our dinner tables. It's a promotional exaggeration from big agriculture that we're feeding the world. That just isn't true.

When we track where the corn goes after harvest when headed to the table, we have to look at the processing journey corn goes through, before it becomes a part of a food product. Corn is processed into glucose, dextrose, high fructose corn syrup and corn sugar and sold to companies that utilize these sweeteners for manufacturing highly processed foods as sweeteners. All major food manu-facturers promote these highly processed food products. In fact, the top 100

---

[7] Custom Query on USDA ERS, Accessed December 2019. https://data.ers.usda.gov/FEED-GRAINS-custom-query.aspx

food companies in America have managed to add more than $61 billion in sales value between them in the last year—an average of $689 million each.[8] These ingredients are then put in cereals, crackers, baked goods, breads, snack foods, sweetened yogurt, ice creams, sodas, etc.

Take a moment right now. Put down your computer or book, walk into your pantry and start reading a food label. Corn is everywhere. Look for those ingredients previously mentioned, glucose, dextrose, high fructose corn syrup, and corn sugar. The reason these companies are continuing to make profits from highly processed foods is because we, as consumers, continue to buy them. The great concern here is, again, that none of these foods support our health. In fact, they're at the source of degradation of our health. Our sugar intake in America has been equated by some health professionals to be the equivalent of alcohol addiction. Until we as consumers understand the power of our food dollars, these companies will continue to thrive.

Was there any great evil intended with the passage of the Farm Bill? I don't believe so. In fact, just the opposite. It was designed to incentivize our farmers to continue to produce food and make a living off the land, but it needs some serious reevaluation of what we should subsidize, if anything, and to whom that money should be provided. No one really knows what would happen if the subsidies stopped tomorrow, but there would likely be unintended consequences, including but not limited to, fewer food-like substances produced in America. The largest and farthest-reaching food system in America has been artificially propped up for the better part of the last hundred years. A slow phase out makes more sense or, at least, gives more consideration for those farmers and ranchers who want to produce food that supports health on smaller diversified vibrant farms all over America.

---

[8] Taylor, K. These 10 Companies Control Everything You Buy, *Business Insider* Sep 28, 2016. https://www.businessinsider. com/10-companies-control-the-food-industry-2016-9#mondelez-5

In addition to the subsidizing of foods, concerns over repeated antitrust lawbreaking across the large-scale conventional agriculture industry causes long-standing damage that sometimes smaller producers cannot recover from. Smaller farmers are routinely driven out of agriculture due to the unequal distribution of the market power. The damage many times is already done via price fixing or gouging before any law enforcement can occur, and, sometimes, the system takes years or decades to react. A quick review of information on topclassactions.com shows price fixing lawsuits in the hundreds of millions being paid out from top meat and dairy conglomerates just in the last few years. My guess is that relative to the profits that were made by domination of the market and the likelihood of being called out on this sort of market overreach, this was just a drop in the bucket and a calculated risk for the industry.

The consistent breach in antitrust laws, in conjunction with a lack of transparency with regards to where our food comes from, keeps the consumer from being able to make an educated choice. It keeps the system disrupted and disconnected. If one wanted to just support American products, it wouldn't be possible. Historically, efforts such as Mandatory Country of Origin Labeling (MCOOL) have been attempted initially through the Tariff Act of 1930. This act required every imported item into this country to disclose the country of origin to the "ultimate purchaser." There are a host of definitions and laws around how far down the food chain a food has to be labeled after it reaches the border and after its modification from its original form. Functionally, this means that the consumer only sees the country of origin if the end product arrives at the border of the United States in its ready to use packaging. Very rarely is this the case.

MCOOL had been revisited in the 2002 farm bill and revised many times since then. It was implemented in 2009 for a time before some loud opposition from Canada and Mexico forced some additional reconsideration around some of the meat products. In 2015, President Obama under pressure from the World Trade Organization removed COOL for beef and pork to keep Mexico and Canada from imposing lawsuits regarding open trade agreements to the tune of approximately one billion dollars. Because MCOOL preferentially supports domestic animal use, the countries to the north and south of us felt that was unfair.

The most recent iteration of legislation around MCOOL in 2016 requires labeling for lamb chicken, goat meat, farm raised and wild caught fish, shellfish, perishable agricultural commodities, macadamia nuts, peanuts, pecans and ginseng. One can imagine how limited this is relative to the ultimate number of products and sheer volume of food products coming into the country. This sort of legislation has had devastating effects on the local beef and pork industry. For example, these industries were singled out in this last go around with Congress, and were perhaps most devastating to the ranchers who really want to raise their animals in a capacity that supports the health of the animal, consumers, and the environment. The argument against MCOOL has most often been that people don't really care where their food is coming from. This trend is changing, however, with great disdain for the industrialized system and its methodology.

Similarly, legislation to require extensive labeling of GMOs was not passed on a federal level until recently. In Chapter 4, the Blind Leading the Blind, I discuss what legislation is allowed. Some states have passed laws that require some labeling for genetically modified foods, plants, or animals, but these laws aren't all encompassing or enforced on a large scale. Some were even passed but then repealed because of Obama's National Bioengineered Food Disclosure Standard (NBFDS) of 2016. It's still unclear how this will all play out. Compliance with the NBFDS should currently be in effect for all food manufacturers, importers, or retail operations large enough to fall under its jurisdiction by the end of 2021. Food manufacturers that produce less than $2,500,000 in sales per year are exempt from having to label GMO or bioengineered foods. How many food manufacturers does this let through the cracks? A health-conscious consumer should be concerned.

In the video example that the USDA has on their website, https://www.youtube.com/watch?v=rxE2FgrZPVs [9] They provide examples of food labels that would be excluded from the ruling that clearly have bioengineered foods in them. Further, they have decided not to define terms that would be useful to understand as a consumer such as "found in nature" or "conventional breeding." This leaves a large leeway for interpretation for the smaller manufacturers, which did quite well during the pandemic. The loophole in the labeling law as well as its interpretation, which is large enough to fit an elephant through, makes the legislation itself just words on paper. As consumers, we really need to start reading the small print.

This is the GPS of our largest food system, and it cannot get us to a healthier place like Vitality. It's not even pointing us in the right direction. If we understood that the GPS has been disabled for a long time or perhaps that we didn't even need the GPS, we might make different decisions with regard to our food choices. Let's bring this issue a little closer to home by looking at state food policy and the food systems that they encourage.

State Policy

Food grown or raised by individual states is also influenced by different economic drivers. Food is big business also known as Big Ag, short for big agriculture. Each individual state has its own resources and economic incentives for what business moves into that state. Here in Missouri, we have lots of farmland, which means lots of grazing space. Lots of grazing space means lots of farm animals and lots of grass and hay. There are all sorts of ways to break down agricultural data but in terms of quantity produced for top crop products, we're the number two in the country for forage hay used for hay or haylage, grass silage, or green chop. We're number four in the country for soybean production used as soybeans and number 11 for corn used as grain. In terms of numbers of livestock,

---

[9] USDA ERS, Overview of National Bioengineered Food Disclosure Standard, December 2020.https://www.youtube.com/watch?v=rxE2FgrZPVs

we're number four on the list for the number of turkeys we produce, number eight for calf and cattle and number nine for broilers and other meat type chickens.[10] The point to this is that food production in Missouri is going to be quite different from food production in Florida or Maine. We have no citrus groves or native lobsters in Missouri, for example.

The industrialized food system is what's called vertically integrated. This means that just a few corporations own most of the proteins and seeds in our country. The concerning part of this is that they're exerting control through policy making that's essentially putting the small family farm out of business.

Bear with me a minute while I talk about some of the politics of Big Agriculture in the state of Missouri. In 2013, the Missouri Legislature passed a law that allows for 289,000 acres or 1% of land to be sold to foreign interests. This was otherwise known as Right to Farm. There are currently over 44,000 acres that have been purchased by foreign countries to date. It's challenging to track how it's all being used, but a portion of it is being turned into Concentrated Animal Feeding Operations otherwise known as CAFOs. CAFOs put animals that would normally roam and forage for what they want to eat, now in confined areas, feeding them usually some form of grain, like corn. This legislation was sold under the premise that it would help to bring jobs to the community and support local food.

Even more recently, in March of 2019, Senate Bill 391 was passed that says that these foreign interests can now move into any county and because of Right to Farm, their interests supersede any county health regulations or zoning regulations that would put restrictions on building these CAFOs. This means that those last 245,000 acres of farmland can be built on essentially unimpeded land, with very limited to no restrictions on CAFOs or how that land is treated. While that may seem appealing on some level to the average freedom-loving American,

---

[10] 2021 Missouri State Agriculture Overview, USDA. https://www.nass.usda.gov/Quick_Stats/Ag_Overview/stateOverview.php?state=MISSOURI

that also means they can do whatever they want to the land, environmentally conscious or not.

To be clear, wherever a CAFO is comes a decrease in property values, contamination of our waterways, and a decrease in overall quality of life when you don't want to walk outside your house because it smells so bad and the air quality has deteriorated. Some studies have shown that the air quality with rates of asthma and respiratory illness are increasing in areas around CAFOs. Health ordinances and zoning regulations directly impact how close a CAFO can be placed to a residence, how big it can be relative to location, how they dispose of waste, even whether they need construction permits and how much they cost. According to a Cornell University blog, 200 cattle creates more waste than a small city of 8,400 people.[11] This isn't something you want in your backyard. There's more to this story that I'll finish in the community section of the chapter, but, essentially, the state of Missouri could be overrun with CAFOs because our legislature allowed for it, despite some very loud opposition.

The additional impact of CAFOs from the health standpoint that gets over-looked routinely is that animals fed in confined spaces are also 1) fed things they wouldn't normally eat, and 2) fed prophylactic antibiotics to keep the animals from getting sick because they're in confined quarters. It has been known since the 1940s that it also allows the animal to grow faster. We are what we eat but we're also what they eat! This impacts the quality of the meat product, as grains decrease Omega 3 fatty acid content of the end product and the antibiotic residues in the meats also disrupt the bacterial flora in our own GI tracts or the human microbiome. Most of our immune system directly functions from our GI tracts. If the microbial flora is thrown off, then we leave ourselves open to an assortment of problems, including autoimmune, gastrointestinal, endocrine, and cardiovascular problems.

---

[11] Phosphorus and the Environment, Setting the Record Straight: Comparing Bodily Waste between Diary Cows and People, June 21, 2017, Cornell University Publication. blogs.cornell.edu/whatscroppingup/2017/06/21

We currently only have approximately 700 registered CAFOs in Missouri. This doesn't account for those that started operations in one classification and then expanded to another without notifying the state regulators.[12] In the state of Iowa, there are more than 7,000 CAFOs and none of their waterways are clean. Missouri has been targeted as the next great option for providing opportunity to Big Ag interests to operate unimpeded.

Positive Policy Impacts

Other states implement laws that support the health of its citizens. In California, Prop 65, otherwise known as The Safe Drinking Water and Toxic Enforcement Act of 1986 protects the state's drinking water sources from being contaminated with chemicals known to cause cancer, birth defects, or other reproductive harm, and requires businesses to inform Californians about exposures to such chemicals. They publish a list of chemicals known to cause cancer or reproductive toxicity and new agents are added to the list as they become known. This is substantial because California has the 6th largest economy in the world, so manufacturers attempt to abide by regulations from this law if possible. Some toxins have been placed on the list and then removed after enough research has come out indicating that it's not a potential cancer-causing agent in humans. Some feel that the law is perhaps too restrictive but so much of our approach to preventative health isn't precautionary. It should be precautionary, though, especially prior to utilizing something on a large consumer scale. Most of our so-called healthcare is actually reactive care after some health crisis has occurred such as with the supplement industry. When reactions occur, sometimes life-threatening reactions, should there not be some sort of safeguard for the consumers prior to this happening? Sick care, not health care, has become a Band-Aid for systemic issues with food.

In other states, food policy councils are attempting initiatives to support local food systems to improve the health of its citizens and economies. Missouri

---

[12] Personal communication with Missouri Coalition for the Environment.

doesn't have a state food policy council, but many others do. Food policy councils are important because they're able to address how food systems operate and address policy changes that support local food systems. Some food policy councils are created from executive government order, but others are grassroots efforts from community and nonprofit organizations. These grassroots organizations are less restricted by the government action that may have otherwise influenced them but then sometimes struggle with creating their own structure and effectiveness due to lack of coordination. Many people think of the word "policy" as limiting, and, in some cases, it can be. If we can think of food policy, however, as something that can also protect us, then it can also ensure that positive changes in regional and local food systems can also be supported.

Maine and Vermont both have very active state Food Policy Councils with many regional and city councils working toward food sovereignty, which have not been created by the government. The Maine Network of Community Food Council (MNCFC) has no formal connection with government but actively "knits together councils across Maine" to where most of the state is currently served by one of the councils. This means that no matter where you live, someone is actively working to ensure that food grown or made in that region is getting to a local customer. Most Maine food councils tend to be rural, which encourages focusing more on direct action than policy. Because there are now twelve local or regional councils, they're doing a design review of their network to better serve the needs of their communities. They have an online mapping tool called the Maine Food Atlas https://mainefoodatlas.org/food-atlas/ that's essentially a visual representation of local food availability and program bases that support local food initiatives and access to food. Much of their efforts are accomplished through curated crowdsourcing rather than governmental or grant funding.

Maine, at the end of 2021, also passed a "right to food" constitutional amendment, the first in the country. People from Maine now have the "natural and unalienable right" to produce, consume, and sell the foods produced on the farm with fewer restrictions. This is an extension of the already existing Cottage Laws, which govern food growth and processing at home in the state and is an example of how deregulation allows for more freedom to live a food sovereign lifestyle. Food sovereignty is basically a food system that allows for the people to control the mechanisms of production and distribution rather than being dictated by the government. It may seem odd that these rights don't already exist, but many of the food laws in this country are based around concerns for food safety and attempting to keep the consumer healthy or without foodborne illness. Sixty percent of folks from Maine supported this constitutional amendment toward the end of the COVID crisis. One might ask themselves whether the increase in food insecurity brought to light how truly dependent we are on a system that didn't deliver.

Vermont Farm to Plate Network https://www.vtfarmtoplate.com/network is housed in a nonprofit entity but was governmentally mandated. This council has members on its board who are government employees, and the government will seek guidance from the council on issues that influence healthy food access, land use, and economic development. They're responsible for implementing the goals of the Vermont Agriculture and Food System Strategic Plan 2021-2030. This plan had over 1,500 people who were vested in the local food system contribute to its development. People who are vested include anyone who relies on the local food system for their vitality. The sheer number of people who were involved in this process shows how this state emphasizes the importance of local food systems to support the jobs of the people doing the hard work of growing food in their state. Their vision was for local food to account for 10% of the state's food dollars by 2020. As of publication, I'm unsure whether they reached their goal!

Another good example that's utilized in many states, including Missouri, would be the Double Up Food Bucks program. The Double Up Food Bucks program doubles the value of SNAP (Food Stamps) dollars spent on locally grown fresh fruits and vegetables. For every dollar spent on local produce at participating farmers' markets and grocery stores in Missouri, Double Up Food Bucks matches a dollar FREE for more fruits and veggies, up to $25 per day. The funding support here in Missouri was supported by Wholesome Wave, a nonprofit organization that supports local and regional food systems as well as the nation's largest prescription program for fruits and vegetables. These state programs are administered on a community level through local farmers' markets.

This increases access to healthy food for folks who may not be able to afford as much otherwise and increases the pull through of the farmers' markets without having to create their own program. There are, of course, some limitations on what the money can be spent on but, overall, a great benefit to consumers with limited income.

Cottage Laws also exist to support local and regional food systems and are passed on a state level. Cottage Laws exist in all states except New Jersey now and allow for nonperishable foods to be produced in a non-certified kitchen. In Missouri, we can produce up to $50,000 worth of revenue off a property. Laws within individual states are different, so be sure to check your state guidelines should you embark on such an endeavor. These laws vary statewide. The common elements according to the 2018 publication from the Food Law Policy Clinic at Harvard Law School on Cottage Food Laws in the United State[13] include: 1) the types of cottage food products allowed; 2) where cottage food products can be sold; 3) required registration, licenses, and/or permits for cottage food operators; 4) how much revenue a cottage food producer can generate before they must move to a commercial facility; 5) required labeling for products produced in a cottage food operation; and 6) tiers or types of cottage food producers, in states that have different rules for different food items or types of cottage food producers.

A much less restrictive version of the Cottage Law is seen in the Food Freedom Laws. An increasing number of states are enacting Food Freedom Laws, which allow for the farmer to sell directly to consumers with much fewer restrictions on food safety as long as the consumer is aware of what they're getting. Wyoming, North Dakota, Illinois and Maine all have versions of Food Freedom Laws that allow for people to have increased autonomy with regard to sales of on-farm food generation in different forms. The most restrictions are placed on foods that would be considered high risk, which includes dairy, meat products,

---

[13] Cottage Food Laws in the United States, Food Law and Policy Clinic, Harvard Law School, August 2018. https://www.chlpi.org/wp-content/uploads/2013/12/FLPC_Cottage-Foods-Report_August-2018.pdf

and canned foods but also vary from state to state. Some might argue that people should have the right to produce food unrestricted and sell what they want, but, on some level, these laws are designed to protect the consumer.

Many of these laws are executed at the community level. Individual farmers' markets have to apply for Double Up Food Bucks and most commonly the enforcement of the food laws fall to the local health departments. Food service permitting, registrations, licenses and inspections are done on county level as well. Some states also require food safety training before or within a certain time frame of starting any food operation, which usually also defaults to the county or community level for administration as well. So, let's walk into the community realm of influence.

Community Policy

When discussing what policy influences our health on a community level, it's almost impossible to have this discussion without first understanding that our health is relative to our immediate external environments, meaning our schools, workplaces, neighborhoods, and communities. The following is taken straight from the Office of Disease Prevention and Health Promotion website:

"We know that taking care of ourselves by eating well and staying active, not smoking, getting the recommended immunizations and screening tests, and seeing a doctor when we are sick all influence our health. Our health is also determined in part by access to social and economic opportunities; the resources and supports available in our homes, neighborhoods, and communities; the quality of our schooling; the safety of our workplaces; the cleanliness of our water, food, and air; and the nature of our social interactions and relationships. The conditions in which we live explain in part why some Americans are healthier than others and why Americans more generally are not as healthy as they could be."

This is otherwise known as social and environmental determinants of health. Have you ever sat down and thought that you would be healthier if there were a grocery store that provided healthy foods within walking distance to your house? Or if there were walking trails close to your apartment complex or home? Community initiatives that support social and physical environments support the health of all. Often, we don't think in these terms when looking for a place to live but these are the things that influence us over the long term. For the purposes of this book, we're going to focus on that which impacts food and our physical environments around food and food systems.

When looking at our external environments, we must also zero in more closely on what's considered a food environment. Our food environment dovetails closely with social determinants of health because they, by definition, consider the same impacts with regard to access to food, proximity to grocery stores, healthy food access and public policy surrounding initiatives to support opportunities for healthy food choices. According to the National Collaborating Center for Environmental Health in their 2015 publication, *Food Environments: An Introduction for Public Health Practice*,[14] "Food environments are created by the human-built and social environments. They are the physical, social, economic, cultural, and political factors that impact the accessibility, availability, and adequacy of food within a community or region." Food environments can also affect what we choose to bring inside our homes as well as whether we are able or decide to cook and sit down and eat with our family that day.

All of these factors affect our daily food choices and, ultimately, our overall health. Unfortunately, we Americans have decided to eat most of our food dollars outside the home. This means that we're no longer in charge of what we're putting into our bodies.

Take a good long hard look around you. Look at your neighborhood. Look at your access to food. Is there a fast-food joint closer than the nearest grocery store? What types of foods does the closest grocery store carry? Is a convenience store closer than the grocery store? How many times have you stopped into the

[14] Rideout, K.,. Mh, C. L., & Minaker, L. Food Environments: An Introduction for Public Health Practice, National Collaborating Center for Environmental Health, December 2015. http://www.ncceh.ca/sites/default/files/Food_Environments_ Public_Health_Practice_Dec_2015.pdf

convenience store, got a quick grab and go for breakfast, filled up the car with a tank of gas, and gone on your way? Does this influence your health? You betcha! This isn't meant as a point of criticism but of notation for what may be affecting decisions around food and consideration for how it's impacting your health. These are the workings of our days that we need to begin to consider in an effort to affect our food environments.

Many people also live in what are called food deserts. Food deserts are areas that lack access to affordable fruits, vegetables, whole grains, and other foods that make up a full and healthy diet. This is defined differently depending upon whether you live in the city or country. Not everyone can run out to the store on a whim and pick up what they need. I recently had an interaction with a patient who had walked 60 miles to get food in rural Missouri. This may be the extreme, but it was the reality of his circumstance. If he had paid for a cab or Uber, he wouldn't have had any money for food.

The most influential policy control is actually at the community level when it comes to food environments. While federal and state policy has a direct impact on what can be accomplished on a community level, communities tend to be more nimble and able to respond more quickly and have the greatest impact on health because it affects us closest to home. Many times, community, county, or city policy trumps state policy as long as it was established before other policy efforts. This means that this is where the rubber meets the road. For those who enjoy or have the desire to influence local environments and engage in community initiatives, this should be encouraging. This also means investing in community in such a way that places an emphasis on the education of our citizens to understand their influence is also important.

A great example of this is New Growth/Deep Roots development in Osceola, Missouri. I recently had an opportunity to sit down with Patty Cantrell, Executive Director, to discuss some of their community development efforts. New Growth/Deep Roots outreaches to a nine-county area that approaches community development not to attract big factories, but to essentially support the rural and innate possibilities of the area that already exist. When we visited, she led me first on a walking tour of Osceola, down to the waterfront and back up around to the center of the square all the while discussing the desire for their community. Patty explained that their approach wasn't driven just by local food initiatives but also with rural living and tourism. By having this multifaceted approach, people may be attracted to the area for one reason but then their overall experience is supported by the other attractions the area has to offer. A report by Travel Trak America 2019[15] highlights that domestic overnight visitors in the state of Missouri spent an average of $104 per person per day, day trippers spent an average $93 per person, and the overall average was $103 per person per day creating $2.48 billion in tax revenue in 2019. Having the long vision and recognizing the tourism potential for Osceola could have long lasting economic influences when actively pursued.

One of their recent initiatives, worked in cooperation with three Chambers of Commerce, helped facilitate the Butterfield Trail connector through to the Frisco Highline trail from the Katy Trail. This effectively would bring offroad mountain biking through Osceola connecting 250 miles of gravel road mountain biking from Springfield to Kansas City or St Louis. In Osceola, there are options for overnight camping next to the Osage River, historical site seeing, and a grocery store as well as a visit to Subway if desired. This is a prime example of how efforts made on a community level affect the quality of life in and around the area by supporting connections of what already exists and by supporting tourism.

New Growth/Deep Roots is also supporting local agricultural efforts, again, that connect people. There have been pockets of people growing their own food as well as some community gardens but, essentially no way to get surplus food coming out of the gardens to the people who need it. Working with and coordinating the community relationships that already exist, they recently obtained some funding from the USDA, to support these grower systems that will then

---

[15] Economic Impact and Visit Characteristics of Tourism in Missouri Fiscal Year 2019 Executive Summary, TravelTrakAmerica, 2019. https://mdt-visitmo-cdn. s3.amazonaws.com/industry-files/OBP-Targeted-And-Nationwide-Markets-FEB-2020/1582739488-economicimpactreportfy2019-executivesummary.pdf

feed into Kansas City markets. Every year, they also have a Farm to Fork Summit aimed at gathering folks for networking opportunities, educational series for young and old, panel workshops, as well as cooking demonstrations.

The idea is that Osceola, Missouri, becomes a destination where people want to live, work, and play. Isn't this what we all want to some degree in our own communities? A place to live and work that we can be proud of and want to come home to?

Zoning Impacts Development

In the most simplistic sense, the way that property is zoned influences what can be accomplished with the property. In general, there are four major zoning classifications: residential, agricultural, commercial, and industrial. A1(Agricultural-1) zoning in one city may have somewhat different criteria for compliance than A-1 zoning in another part of the country. Every parcel of land in America has a zoning classification. In addition to zoning classifications, the development of some parcels of land are also governed by special procedures and planned districts. So, for instance, you may have a great idea that you're going to put a large garden on your residential property and sell food out of your yard but there may be other restrictions that the city may have in place that won't allow this. They may want you to rezone your property and/or put in additional support for the built environment on your property, such as a parking lot for your customers. Please remember also, that just because something has been put in print with regard to zoning doesn't mean that a city will allow you to do what's written into the zoning designation with your property.

Similarly, a local food policy council may have some great initiatives for identifying lots in and around a city that could be used for community gardens. If working with the city, this initiative would have less pushback on zoning and rezoning if the city supported and understood the importance and benefits for using these spaces in this capacity. Empty buildings for small supermarkets placed in underserved neighborhoods would be another example. So, education, even for City governments, is sometimes in order. And just because education occurs, doesn't mean cooperation will follow.

Unfortunately, most zoning isn't necessarily approved with sustainability in mind. While there's usually a rigorous process associated with it, it really depends on the mindset of the leadership within each individual community as well as the community itself, and much of it is financially driven. Some of the cities, like Madison, Wisconsin, that have strong sustainability initiatives provide great examples of how local food can also be incorporated within the development of the city. The mayor's office website has a full page dedicated to food in the city with links and access to the many food programs in and around the city, including community gardens, food access improvement maps, healthy retail access programs, edible landscaping permits, Double-Up Food Bucks, healthy food retail and underserved neighborhoods, summer food programs, and more. The impressive more recent work involving the offering of grant funds from money was legislated to be reallocated for Community Food Access Grants when COVID-19 hit. The Madison Food Policy Council was advocating for folks to apply for these $25,000 individual grants that support the local food system that increased access to healthy food for Madison citizens.

Many other cities, however, are fortunate if they just have a recycling program. "Sustainability most often cannot be achieved without a complete overhaul of most communities' policies." This quote from the Sustainable Development Code Project which is a best-practice website for anyone interested in making development codes in their community more sustainable. Chapter 6.2 of the code addresses issues around food insecurity and provides best practice guidelines for removing code barriers, providing incentives and filling in regulatory gaps to move cities toward a more sustainable environment that supports the health of its citizens, https://sustainablecitycode.org/chapter/chapter-6/6-2/. Codes and zoning are derived from the mindset of the people making the policies. In most cases, these are elected officials. If not elected, they may be working for an elected official. Don't forget that as elected officials, they should be working for you. Don't be afraid to speak up with questions or concerns that you have in your community.

The CAFO Disconnect

Many times, we as citizens of a community are unaware of the connections between what's read in the newspaper or heard about on the news relative to what we do in our daily lives. Recently, I had an opportunity to be engaged in a community effort to bring awareness to a statewide initiative focused on bringing CAFOs to our state unimpeded. The efforts were trying to be accomplished via an initiative under Missouri Farm Care called AgriReady. Missouri Farm Care is a front for large agribusiness such as Monsanto, Cattleman's Association, and other Big Ag efforts. In order for a county to be AgriReady, the county has put in an application to have their local ordinances to be reviewed for any limitations to CAFOs operating within the county. The presentation to the county commissioners is that the county would be open to supporting agriculture as an opportunity for local, economic income.

On the surface, it sounds supportive of local agriculture, but below the surface, AgriReady was a beacon for letting Big Ag interests know that the county has no ordinances in place that would keep them from operating unimpeded. In Christian County, where I lived, we had no ordinances to keep CAFOs from operating unimpeded, so we scrambled to have a Health Ordinance instituted that would keep Big Ag interests from coming into our county and purchasing agriculturally zoned land to be used for this purpose. Many counties in our state were able to get Health Ordinances passed, but in Christian County, we weren't able to accomplish this. Had we been successful, this would be an example of county policy designed to mitigate damage from state policy.

The unfortunate reality is that a consistent misrepresentation of information and a creeping in of policy changes allow Big Ag to be successful with these endeavors. The information is objectively accurate from the financial perspective but not inclusive of the ultimate results, which include decrease in property values, poor water and air quality, money that doesn't stay in our state, and increased production of environmentally unconscious unhealthy food right outside our back doors. In this case, the "Right to Farm" coupled with the Missouri legislature allowing for farmland to be purchased by foreign entities, and then the passage of SB 391 in Missouri ensured that CAFOs would thrive in our state. Unlike a regenerative, locally owned farm with a vested interest in maintaining the relationships fostered locally, a CAFO mainly creates economic opportunities only for the people that own them. The policy damage here doesn't appear to be reversible.

What does that mean for our county? Besides supporting the increased availability of unhealthy meat products, perhaps the greatest impact will be when our citizens want to enjoy the semi- unimpaired waterways that currently exist in our state. Tourism is a $17.9 billion industry in Missouri. Not only our own citizens but people come here to vacation at the local and scenic riverways and lakes. Gradually, our waterways will become overgrown, most commonly, with E. coli and algae blooms from the increase in manure waste and fertilizer runoff that finds its way into our waterways because of poorly managed agricultural land. They'll no longer be a destination for our people because they'll no longer have enough clean water to enjoy. People generally don't frequent mucky water. We need to have a symbiotic relationship with the earth and, in this case, taking care of our health means taking care of how our local farms and land are treated. Remember too, everybody lives downstream. This means that the two rivers that run through our county, the James and Finley rivers, will then be taking the waste from any CAFO development to the next county downstream and ultimately to the ocean in the Gulf of Mexico.

Policy for the People

While this is an example of a negative environmental impact there are other policy-related community initiatives that can have a positive impact on access to healthy foods. Some of these include whether a school system has a Farm to School initiative or a school garden to teach children about growing food. School and Community Gardens are fantastic ways to draw in people to learn more and reconnect with food and the soil.

Local businesses and institutions can also have internal policies that influence on a community level as well. Health Care Without Harm business initiatives frequently involve supporting local and regional food systems. "Our Healthy Food in Health Care program harnesses the purchasing power, expertise, and voice of the healthcare sector to advance the development of a sustainable food system."[16] The purchasing power of a larger business or hospital, if a smaller local producer can meet demand, will frequently be the anchor for that business if the relationship remains beneficial to one another. Anchor institutions provide consistent business pull-through of products to ensure that the farmer has a place to sell their product the next year. This is what helps to build the local food economy.

Some communities have seed-saving efforts. While this may not be a written policy, seed saving efforts, despite the low cost of initiating such an effort, can have a significant impact on community relationship building as well as empowering people to understand how to grow their own food. I recently had an opportunity to hear Ben Cohen http://www.smallhousefarm.com/about-us/ speak at one of our local seed festivals at Baker Creek Seed Company. He makes a strong case for saving the most resilient Heirloom seeds from our crops because heirloom, old world seeds are able to be planted over and over again to produce food. This is important because most seeds produced in America don't have this capability anymore. Heirloom seeds are old world seeds that have not been genetically modified or hybridized and can reseed themselves. He even selects for the most resilient seeds that make it through a hard winter.

Additionally, there are also plenty of producers who don't sell at farmers' markets. Farmers' markets should be considered interim market opportunities for producers. Some don't want to be taken off the farm for half a day and pay the expense of the market. Some promote their products on national websites such as www.localharvest.org instead. Don't be afraid to reach out to your neighbor and ask if they're selling or would be willing to sell their products. Have a conversation

---

[16] Healthcare Without Harm Website. https://noharm-uscanada.org/issues/us-canada/healthy-food-health-care

with your neighbor about how they manage their chickens running around the yard and if they would be willing to sell some eggs to you. Many times, the people around the corner or over the hill down yonder are producing high quality food products pretty close to home. These are the interactions that support your health socially as well as physically. While they may not have a written policy around how they manage their farm, many producers grow and raise their own food because of concerns they have about the industrialized food system.

Many regions have food policy councils that are also looking at supporting food initiatives on a local level relative to identified needs. As previously mentioned, in 2013, in Springfield, MO, we launched the Ozarks Regional Food Policy Council (ORFPC) and the first food system assessment ever accomplished within the region. The document that was produced from the food system assessment identified some deficits within our region, and many organizations vested in the food system launched additional effort and applied for grant support around those identified needs. The ORFPC now functions as the Food Collaborative at Community Partnership of the Ozarks and continues to support community food system initiatives.

Targeted food system assessments are useful because they identify the wants, needs, desires, and deficits of a local food system. They bring together like-minded people who want to support the built environment and develop or coordinate programs that support the food system or ensure that policy that supports these endeavors exists. Sometimes, it can be as simple as mapping existing food-related services, having a city change bus routes for greater access to grocery stores, encouraging governmental agencies to purchase from local producers, or helping to coordinate local markets. The needs within an area will be different relative to the existing built environment, housing issues, and identified community needs.

While we see some of the social determinants of health and our food environments' influence on the community level, perhaps the greatest effect is on the personal level. Not everyone has an opportunity to sell their house for a better location, but we all have conscious decisions that we can make every day that influence our most immediate food environments: our homes.

Personal Policy

So, let's think about this for just a minute. If our national policy allows for large-scale availability of subsidized unhealthy food to be available for us and our state policy, in many cases, also allows for unhealthy food products, the degradation of policy in our rural communities and environmental hazards brings it even closer to home. Our community policy pretty much dictates the food environment when we step outside our homes. Shouldn't we have a personal policy around food choices and the creation of food environments in our homes? This is one of the few things that's totally in our charge regardless of all other policies.

This sounds pretty formal. "Personal food policy." Nothing would make me happier than to hear every child across the country talk about what they believe about food, how and why they choose what they eat. Sounds a little crazy, doesn't it? Every child in America knows what the golden arches are though, right? A huge paradigm shift needs to occur in our homes. What if every child in kindergarten could articulate on some level that their body is their temple and they wanted to put good wholesome fuel into it every day? This is perhaps a pipe dream of mine.

We're busy, very busy, as a society and as individuals. This busy-ness has created a culture of convenience in America that leaves us headed to the golden arches feeding hungry bellies rather than choosing healthy food options. While food trends indicate that people are becoming more interested in supporting the environment and making more mindful decisions about what we're choosing to put in our bodies, we still eat out too much and aren't choosing well as evidenced by our health statistics and the thriving of those junk food companies mentioned previously. According to the USDA ERS, we eat 54% of our food dollars outside the home. National consumption patterns show that we eat far too few vegetables and that only one in 10 people are getting enough.[17] Current recommendations from the American Cancer Society are to consume six to nine servings of fruits or vegetables per day. The serving size is one half cup if it's cooked and one cup if it's raw. Pay attention for a few days. Write it down. How many servings do you eat a day? Ask yourself why you only eat that few. In my experience, the number one cited reason has and will always be, I don't have time. Are we really that busy or do we just think we are?

Just to humor myself one day, I timed how long it took me to boil a free-range egg from a local farmer, sauté some vegetables, cook some toast and slather it with grass-fed butter. Most of the time was spent boiling the egg. That process took 12 minutes total which I significantly diminished that time by cooking many eggs in advance so the process then only lasted two minutes. Guess how much time the average person spends sitting in a drive though? According to QSR, in 2021, the average time was 4.4 minutes or 264 seconds to be exact.[18] This drive through time is down almost an entire minute from 2019. I can assure you that many fast-food restaurants aren't that fast, however. To humor myself further, I sat out at the Taco Bell down the hill from my house during lunch to see how long it took from getting in line to receiving a meal and the average was 6 minutes. And this didn't include travel to and from the restaurant. At home, however, we can eat breakfast together, talk about what we had planned that day and sometimes we even get the dishes done in another three to four minutes. Fifteen minutes is the total time for a sit-down breakfast that leaves everyone feeling a little more settled for the day, and it's actually less expensive and time consuming. Our whole meal was under a dollar, and we made healthy food choices because we knew what we were eating. This act of cooking and eating at

---

[17] CDC Newsroom, Only 1 in 10 Adults Gets Enough Fruits and Vegetables, November 16, 2017. https://www.cdc.gov/media/releases/2017/p1116-fruit-vegetable-consumption.html

[18] QSR 2022 The Drive Through Report, Danny Klein, October 2022. https://www.qsrmagazine.com/reports/2022-qsr-drive-thru-report

home is lost in America but, foundationally, this behavior needs to be incorporated again before we Americans can regain our health.

The number one most consumed food in America is the hamburger followed closely by the pizza. This wouldn't be as concerning if most of the beef on our tables were high-quality grass-fed beef. I consider grass-fed beef a healthy food because the Omega 3 content of the meat product is higher than conventionally raised meat. Otherwise, industrialized beef should be considered proinflammatory and not something to eat routinely. Cows fed corn and held in those confined areas we previously discussed shouldn't be eaten, yet it's the number one food in America. Pizza has the same problem. That supreme pizza topped with four industrial raised meat products, only a quarter cup of vegetables, and a huge list of additives and preservatives is no better for you.

In 2014, I started Remo's Mobile Pizzeria. The logo for the trailer is our family farm dog Remo, and the tagline is Wood Fired/Locally Sourced. The logo speaks to our personal food policy. Remo's was started due to my passion for food and being a dietitian; this is my version of some of the healthiest fast food I could provide that people would eat on a large scale. All the meat toppings are sourced year-round from local producers who support the community and raise their animals with at least some sustainable agricultural practices. For a while, we were raising most of the ground beef and lamb toppings ourselves. Vegetable toppings were sourced locally when in season from farmers who support regenerative agriculture or from what we would grow ourselves. If there's no line, it takes about four minutes from the time you order your pizza to the time the pizza is handed to you. This is our version of fast food. Do we occasionally have to make substitutions due to unavailability? Of course. But our policy is to support the local farmer who's trying to make a difference with their agricultural practices.

I realize that not everyone has the resources or motivation to start their own pizzeria, but we all have some resources. Most everyone has the option to eat at home, to grocery shop, to cook, to grow food in some capacity. What are you willing to do differently today that will support your health instead of the food system that's currently degrading our health? I have some additional thoughts and ideas in Chapter 8 that encourage healthier food choices. Remember that our personal food policy affects not only health and well-being but also influences all other systems mentioned. Our personal food policies dictate how we interact with the community as well as whether we're supporting the environment. Food is so much more than just something to keep us from being hungry or nourishing our bodies. It's a portion of the very foundation of our community base when offered with sustainability in mind. If you frequent the local farmers' market with any regularity, you'll begin to experience what I mean by this.

My personal policy is to eat at home as much as possible. It's also to support my local farmers and friends who are practicing regenerative organic agriculture. Also, I grow as much of my own food in this manner as well. This means that I can take as much charge as possible about what goes into my body, and my knowledge base for how to do this is ever expanding. Initially, I had a lot of questions, but, just like anything, the more you do something, the easier it gets. Does this mean that I never eat out? Of course, I do, but I'm very careful about where and purposefully support restaurants that support local producers in an effort to support the local food system. Start having conversations with your friends about farm-to-table restaurants and where they are in your location. A quick internet search will provide you with a variety of options. Even when you travel, search for farm-to-table eateries to stop at along the way. Just remember that this is your ultimate food environment where you exhibit your own food policy: home.

3.
How About a Compass Instead of GPS.

If one were to search for food systems graphics, there would be a variety of confusing graphs, with arrows pointing all over the place that would make even the most astute scholar want to shake their head and run in the other direction. For the purpose of understanding as well as simplification for this book, I like to depict the food system as a compass. While this is an oversimplification when viewing our current food system, because the cross currents in those graphics are quite importantly intertwined, it helps to narrow the focus toward simplicity for fundamental understanding. At the center of the compass is the vibrant, regenerative farm. Surrounding this vibrant farm are the north, south, east, and west arms of the compass. The arms include healthy people, strong communities, regenerative ecosystems, and thriving local economies.

The reason that the local vibrant farms are at the center is because without the farm and its ability to support the other arms, there's no local food system. All the other arms could survive on a cursory level in some capacity without the vibrant farm at its center but only on a service level. This is evidenced by what's currently occurring in and around American rural communities, but the small vibrant farm has multiple purposes. It supports multiple bottom lines. It provides healthy food, picked at the peak of ripeness for its citizens and supports the local ecosystem when these foods are raised regeneratively. The local economy thrives not only because folks are buying from the farm but also because the farm is supporting their individual business endeavors, and relationships are built over time that continuously pull the community together.

While this may seem like a pipe dream to some, it's absolutely essential that we get back to supporting our small local vibrant regenerative farms. The misunderstanding that we need genetically modified food and large CAFOs to feed the world needs to be purposefully reconsidered. All it has done is helped to centralize our food system, made a few people quite wealthy, and left most people with access to mostly unhealthy food and lives all while impairing our ecosystem. The paradigm shift needs to bring money back to our own Vitality, which creates fresh local food but supports a local community and economy as well as the health of its citizens and ecosystem. Let's break the compass down further by defining the Vibrant Farm and its individual arms to look at this more closely.

What's a Vibrant Farm?

This description should sound somewhat familiar as it was provided also at the beginning of the book as well as through examples throughout the book. There, we called the fictitious regenerative farm Vitality. Vitality supports its own ecosystem, builds its own local supply chains, uses regenerative organic agricultural practices, pays a fair wage for services provided as well as treats workers fairly. Without the center of the compass, all else defaults back to the industrialized food system and ways of doing things where it's no longer about relationships and supporting a local food economy.

Vitality is where people, the environment, our health, and local economies can thrive and are all of tantamount importance. It's done with a purpose. This is the place where ancillary businesses are created because the farm exists here. This is the place where a business owner started a farm-to-table restaurant because of a relationship he had with the owners of the local farms, and most people know each other. This is a place where people lead "food-centric" lives. That's to say, people's lives are centered around food and all of its ancillary influences.

Hypothetically, the local ice cream shop gets its milk from that local Vitality dairy and creates fun flavors of ice cream like lemon lavender from herbs and fruit harvested from another local farm. This is the place where people walk to the honor system farmstand down the street to get fresh fruits and vegetables for their dinner that evening, and they stop to share recipes because others are doing the same thing. The honor system works here because everyone knows that there are times when folks can give more and understand that hard times occur and, sometimes, they give less. This is a place where, when there's a crisis, food costs remain relatively stable. This is a place where the community comes together when there's great need, and where people live at ease because no one wonders where their next meal comes from. People find a way to make things work by coming together as a community because not only are people their greatest resource, but this is the way they've always done it, as community has been their biggest priority.

The only form of agriculture that's practiced on and around this farm is regenerative organic. The reason for this is that the founders of vibrant farms understand that how they treat their land impacts not only their health as owners and their neighbors but the environment as well. The quality of the food is impacted because regenerative management of the soil allows for the biology in the soil to support the nutrient availability of what's in the soil for the plant. This translates into more nutrition for the plant as well as the people eating it! This symbiosis is found often in nature when on-farm operations are working with nature rather than against her.

This same symbiosis can be found with the bees. Bees touch one out of every three bites of our food. This means that without them, we wouldn't be eating much. One might hypothesize that if you're vegetarian, it might be two out of every three bites. Our ecosystems will fail without them. Vibrant farms should include their own bees, if possible, to ensure that their crops are pollinated close to home, keeping them from being influenced by potential pesticide residues from outside their local habitat.

This is where almost everything you need for longevity is at your fingertips, so a handheld non-digital compass rather than a GPS is all that's needed. People are healthier here because they're supported, eat fresh local regeneratively grown and raised food, take fewer medications, and know that the community comes together in times of great need.

Healthy People Arm

Vibrant farms produce healthy food options that, in turn, support healthy people. Think back to before the industrialization of our food supply. We ate what was available to us at the time. Refrigeration didn't become mainstream until the 1930s, so prior to that time, if there was surplus from a backyard garden, it was either shared with a neighbor or turned into a more shelf-stable product via fermentation, canning or drying. Many times, people gathered together to accomplish this so there was a large degree of socialization and hard work around these food events. Here in Missouri, there used to be over 100 tomato canneries, as this was a great place to grow tomatoes. Sadly, there are now no tomato canneries, and this fact is just part of our displaced food history. Many of the old stone cannery buildings still stand, empty on roadsides all over the state. Some years, there were even crop failures due to drought, blight, or natural disasters. This meant folks just did without certain foods.

We also ate seasonally, rather than having a constant availability of all foods. In functional nutrition circles this is known as ancestral eating patterns. Don't get me wrong, it's great to have mangos and avocados available all year long, but we don't grow mangos or avocados in Missouri. To have them any time of year should be considered a delicacy but it isn't anymore. It's expected. The average consumer is quite spoiled by the land of opportunity and the industrialized food system whereby we can get whatever food we want when we want it. Sometimes, I have to remind myself of this when I cannot find a ripe avocado or mango in January for a food preparation demonstration.

Let's think through this for just a moment. What if there's a reason why there are seasons for food? What if our bodies need a break from even healthy foods? What if cycling in and out of healthy foods relative to season and location had a purpose behind it? This is known as an ancestral eating pattern. Let's use blackberries in Missouri as an example. The native blackberry season in Missouri runs from June through early September. These little morsels are packed with high antioxidant phytochemicals known as phenolic compounds, such as flavonoids, flavanols, and proanthocyanins, that help our bodies manage oxidative stress.

In the middle of the winter, one can drive to the grocery store and pick up some blackberries from somewhere else, some other country usually. It will cost a lot more, but they're certainly available.

What's generally not publicized is that blackberries also contain a lot of oxalates. Oxalates are compounds found in many foods that are high in these phenolic compounds that dietitians consistently recommend eating more of because of their antioxidant, disease reducing potential. Great examples of foods high in oxalates besides blackberries include sweet potatoes, spinach, Swiss chard, most kinds of nuts, rhubarb, beets, chocolate, and star fruit. Under most circumstances, having the opportunity to eat more of these foods year-round would be considered beneficial. But what if you're someone who doesn't metabolize oxalates well? If you're one of these people, the oxalates are drawn into your bloodstream as opposed to being excreted and then deposited in the soft tissues in your body. Calcium chelates or binds to oxalates and helps to pull them through the digestive system without being absorbed. So, those raw spinach (also high in oxalates) and berry smoothies for folks sensitive to this, on the ever trendy gluten free, dairy free diets might find it detrimental rather than supportive of health. Studies suggest that this can be the cause of some of the nondescript pain syndromes like fibromyalgia. If you're one of these people, the dedication to eating these foods year-round because of the industrialized food system could be part of the problem particularly with low calcium intakes.

Another example of health and nutrition that may benefit from ancestral eating patterns is with people who have thyroid concerns. These folks may need to eat limited amounts of raw cruciferous vegetables or soy products. The reason for this is that they're goitrogens. Since the 1920s, it has been known that goitrogens interfere with the normal functioning of the thyroid gland. Cruciferous vegetables include vegetables such as brussels sprouts, kale, cauliflower, broccoli, and cabbage and are all goitrogens. Cooking these foods diminish the goitrogenic effect so the recommendation for folks with thyroid dysfunction is to cook these wonderful detoxifying high sulfur containing foods before eating them if you have thyroid dysfunction or iodine deficiency. And routine raw kale smoothies would certainly not be your friend, despite kale being promoted as a superfood.

Cruciferous vegetables are crops that are normally grown in the cooler time of the year. Ever notice that there isn't any broccoli at the farmer' market in August? But yet we eat it year-round.

Cycling in and out foods from the diet relative to season makes some sense with what we know about food. I cater the nutrition advice to these people to ensure that they eat them cooked because there are so many other benefits to eating them consistently including the antioxidant benefit as well as their prebiotic and detoxifying effect. So again, if we recommend eating just raw food, we would be missing the boat for the ever increasing portion of the population that struggles with thyroid problems.

No Downside to Eating Clean

There really is no one size fits all meal plan for anyone. Everyone's genetics are different, but if there were a single place to start, the research indicates that the Mediterranean Diet (MD) would be that place. The Mediterranean Diet's claim to fame is that it's mostly plant based; most of your plate should be vegetables with a moderate amount of healthy, unprocessed meat, fruit, healthy fats, and a smidgen of grains and dairy on occasion. The preference for meat products would be animals raised in their natural environments. After all, we are what we eat as well as what they eat. And, the MD is noted for high amounts of monounsaturated fat intake from plants like olives, olive oil, avocado and avocado oil, and an assortment of nuts. MDs have consistently been shown to reduce cardiovascular disease as well as all causes of mortality. Any dietitian will tell you that it's a great place to start but, as we age, we may need to cater to what comes up with regard to health that requires specific food interventions and fine tuning relative to our individual circumstances.

Everyone can benefit from clean eating, however. Clean eating essentially means just eating real food. No additives, preservatives, antibiotics, hormones, coloring, or extra junk in our food. When looking at the healthiest pockets of people around the world, they eat clean. They have very few additives added to food for preservation, and they have a dedication to continuing to eat this way.

Pockets of people around the world who live to be the oldest and in good health are prime examples of people who die of "old age." Many of these communities produce most of their own food and stay quite active doing it. Dan Buettner wrote *The Blue Zone Solution* in 2012[19], which brought much attention to the habits around these populations: Ikaria, Greece; Okinawa, Japan; Sardinia, Italy; Loma Linda, California; Nicoya Peninsula, Costa Rica. Interestingly, all of these areas are somewhat isolated or insulated from the outside world because of location or cultural belief. Loma Linda, is the only city that's located in the United States and its numbers are driven by a pocket of approximately 9,000 Adventists living in the area who don't drink alcohol, smoke, or eat meat of any sort. Pesco-vegetarians or the part of the community that eats fish within that community, actually live slightly longer.

Similarities within each region that are noteworthy with regard to diet include according to the Blue Zones website:

1. Stop eating when 80% full.

2. Eat the smallest meal of the day in the evening.

3. Eat mostly plants, limit meat products to 3-4 ounces five times per month.

4. Modest alcohol intakes to fewer than one or two drinks per day.

Each community has their own specialty products or foods, but in each location, they mainly eat what's available within the region. From a nutritional standpoint, these communities raise animals and grow food in accordance with our definitions of the previously defined Vibrant farming community. They eat very limited amounts of meat and dairy but when they do they are not highly processed foods. Many of the animals are raised on grass which optimizes the benefits of Omega- 3 fatty acids in these products and communities with access

---

[19] Buettner, D. *The Blue Zones*, 2012.

to fishing incorporate some fish into the diet, also high in Omega-3 fatty acids. Some animals will also qualify as A2, such as goat and sheep milk, which has an additional level of anti-inflammatory benefit.

All dairy products on the planet can essentially be categorized as A1 or A2. The overwhelming majority of dairy products in America are A1 milk products. This is a concern because A1 milk products pose an additional worry with regard to inflammatory or disease-causing potential in the body due to the type of beta-casein protein within the milk called BCM-7. BCM-7 is the opioid-like beta casein in A1 milk that when it cleaves and enters the bloodstream may facilitate higher rates of type 1 diabetes, heart disease, autism, and mental health disorders.[20] It's believed that, originally, most milk products in America were from A2 animals. Over hundreds of years with the introduction of different breeds of cattle as well as possible genetic mutations, this has changed. Some breeds of cattle, such as Guernsey, Jersey, Charlais, and other Asian herds are more likely to be A2 as well as all sheep and goats This is important because if our farms are raising a grass-fed A2 animal that's also being milked, then this is a superior nutritional quality, less inflammatory product than an A1 animal fed corn with lots of antibiotics. Smaller vibrant farming communities understand the value of managing animals holistically for the health of its citizens as well as the environment.

In the community subheading in Chapter 2, we talked briefly about social determinants of health. The blue zone communities have something that's perhaps just as important as access to healthy food, living close to a grocery store, educational opportunities, or access to walking trails. They have community. COVID has shown us that the lack of socialization can impact our health perhaps more than even eating poorly. A healthy community shows the people that all the members of the communities are valued in their own right. They work together, farm together, live together, and eat together. These strong bonds support all members through the lifespan from birth until old age. This socialization is so

---

[20] Wolford, K. *Devil in the Milk*, 2009.

important for our health and wellness, but it's also what contributes to strong communities. Communities that build lives together, stay together.

Strong Communities

If one looks at definitions of a strong community, it almost always involves a shared sense of purpose and relevance that's interwoven into the fabric of the lives of people within that community. That purpose can really be about anything: raising healthy children, race, an affiliation, gender, career, religion, or even a place like a bar or a region. What makes it a good community also includes membership, either formal or informal, and fulfillment of needs, which influences a shared emotional connection. Strong communities build something called social capital which is the networks of relationships among people who live and work within these communities that allow them to function effectively. For the purposes of this book, it's discussed in terms of local food being the shared purpose. To be clear, sometimes, these networks of relationships start in other places but then extend into the local food arena based on need or desire.

When explaining how local food brings communities together, it's almost easier to provide examples because, unless personally experienced, it's just words on paper. If we view people as our greatest asset, then people are who or what needs to be supported in any organization to ensure its success. Sadly, many times, we separate people or communities from the success endpoint of the organization and define success only by metrics of monetary value.

Community gardens within individual communities are a fantastic way to connect people. I recently had an opportunity to sit down and talk with Dr. John Harms, professor of Sociology at Missouri State University and Dr. Ximena Uribe-Zarain, an ethnographer, to talk about their research on community gardens. The focus of their research was the social capital built around Springfield Community Gardens in Springfield, Missouri. They have held between 10-15 interviews with key contributors to discuss the social capital built around these gardens.

The story behind the gardens goes a bit like this. In 2010, two women, Maile Middlemas-Auterson and Shelley Vaughine along with other community members started an initiative to grow food in a single community garden. Their initial volunteering efforts (Maile 40 hours a week for 7 years!), have now expanded to over 20 gardens around the city that have become what's known as Springfield Community Gardens (SCG). Their efforts were met with some resistance and skepticism, but the ideals of the community garden ultimately won over not just the community but local government and began down this path of incorporating large institutions into the fold. People within the neighborhoods of these gardens even began volunteering for some additional produce. Initially, the organizational structure was a bit loose but became more established and more organized to where Springfield Community Gardens is now a 501c3 nonprofit with a full governing board to help direct its activities. Maile, to this day, remains the current Executive Director of SCG.

These efforts drew the attention of Harms and Uribe-Zarain to learn more about the social capital that has been built around the gardens. According to Harms, social capital requires two things: trust and reciprocity. Trust must precede reciprocity. Reciprocity is the practice of exchanging things with others for mutual benefit. In social psychology, reciprocity is a social norm of responding to a positive action with another positive action, rewarding in kind actions. This can also extend itself to the provision of help with volunteerism, sharing resources and gifting of needed items such as tractors, trailers, and seeds. These resources for the gardens are shared by public and private partnerships that are so important for the Asset Based Community Development (ABCD) that allows these sorts of programs to thrive.

ABCD is a means for communities to develop sustainable action plans based on their strengths and potentials. It involves assessing and accessing the resources, skills, and experience available in a community as well as organizing the community around issues that move its members into action. It empowers community members by encouraging them to utilize resources already available to them, build relationships and trust, and work with one another toward common goals. Essentially, it asks community members to connect the dots with other community members from different backgrounds and come up with solutions to identified needs and problems. In the case of Springfield Community Gardens, the community identified a need for more fresh healthy food in the middle of a low-income/low-access area or food desert in Springfield, Missouri. The support from the community, at first, was slow, but, in recent years, the support has expanded to include grant funding, which requires these relationships for the application, to the tune of greater than $2,000,000 this past year. This funding now supports paid positions, educational outreach, and a program base that feeds and provides opportunities for any resident in Greene County to learn to grow food.

Why have the gardens been so successful? Dr. Harms believes that part of this success can be attributed to the fact that despite how political food is, eating is a nonpartisan issue. Everyone has to eat. If you go to his Food in Society class, he greets every class with, "Good morning fellow eaters!" And it's true, 10 out of 10 people have to eat, which makes his greeting so fun but also accurate. Sociological ties or social capital are formed by all people around the issue of food because of this reason. Social "bonding" is formed between people who are from similar backgrounds and sociological statuses, and we all visit with people who are like us every day, at lunch, in the office, or at an event down the street. But Harms and Uribe-Zarain's research has found that there's strong sociological "bridging" that also develops between people of different sociological backgrounds. In short, community gardens have the ability to bring different people together, regardless of politics or any other agenda, who normally wouldn't associate.

SCG has also expanded outreach to CoxHealth to further some of their initiatives. CoxHealth is one of the largest health systems in SW Missouri. They employ over 12,000 people and continue to grow in hospital numbers and clinic outreach. CoxHealth was willing to partner with SCG for several reasons. SCG's track record of success with the gardens certainly played in their favor.

The first reason for SCG's success is that the community outreach utilizes existing resources. CoxHealth has a large, older kitchen at their north hospital three-fourths of which wasn't being used. SCG had a need for kitchen space to start using and processing some of their produce for "value added" products. "Value added" means, according to the USDA, a change in the physical state or form of the product. The change in physical form of a product usually enhances its value. For us lay people, it means they wanted to turn tomatoes into salsa or veggies and eggs into quiche and sell it for more money. And this is what SCG did. They had been selling farm fresh quiche from the north kitchen at CoxHealth pre-COVID, have a hospital farm that runs a CSA for the employees, and are working to address low-income patients by providing healthy food prescriptions. Sounds simple but this deal was over a decade in the making before it came to fruition. This ABCD example of a public, nonprofit partnership that supports a local food system shows what can be done when specific needs are identified and persistently worked through.

The second reason is that there's a serious shortage of fresh, sustainably raised produce available to large institutions. Recall the discussion about the enhanced nutritional value of foods that are raised regeneratively? SCG is partnering with CoxHealth to produce Certified Naturally Grown food on a three-acre lot across the street from Cox South, their largest hospital with 700 plus beds. Under the Certified Naturally Grown (CNG) designation, CNG farmers don't use any synthetic herbicides, pesticides, fertilizers, or genetically modified organisms. The gardens, with high tunnels, will help to fill a gap for the hospital that, to this day, has attempted to source food locally but, much to their dismay, have not been able to achieve consistently.

I had an opportunity to sit down with Jason Bauer, Director of Food Services at CoxHealth, to discuss his efforts to source locally as well as working through the caveats of a hospital as large as CoxHealth to support local food initiatives. Jason has been dedicated to supporting the small local producer because he understands the value of supporting local and regional food systems in order to support the health of our communities, but, for various reasons, something always happens. Examples of reasons for failure include producers going out of business, producers not wanting to get vaccinations to enter the facility because they don't believe in them, and not following through with filling out forms.

One of the local milk producers even went so far as to have the nutritional analysis of his milk analyzed to prove it was a healthier food product than the average milk on the grocery store shelf. It was certainly higher in Omega 3 Fatty Acids than conventional milk but when it came down to delivering the product in the containers needed and the creation of a value-added product called yogurt, the middle man wanted too much of a cut. It didn't make sense for the local milk producer to continue to try to deliver to CoxHealth. Ultimately and sadly, this milk producer went out of the dairy business for good. He was tired of fighting the good fight.

Springfield Community Gardens (SCG), as a portion of their grant funding efforts, has included support for local and regional food systems as well as teaching other people or potential farmers how to produce their own food regeneratively. The first year of their grant funding includes the startup of Community Supported Agriculture (CSA) for the employees of CoxHealth as well as building a network for selling into local restaurants. As previously discussed, the small local producer generally doesn't have the same funding available to them, so offering programs such as what SCG's Farm Incubator Program, is a significant service to the community that has the potential to provide opportunities for people to become more self-sufficient with their food. Very few farms can make it on their own without some form of policy or additional inputs that support their endeavors.

SCG's efforts epitomize the essence of the strong community whereby people from different backgrounds come together and recognize that they're better working together toward common shared goals rather than attempting to do it alone. These sorts of community initiatives CANNOT be accomplished alone. When local food initiatives also incorporate a component of being cognizant of the impact of our agricultural methods as well, we also have the opportunity to ensure that we're taking only from the earth what we need, supporting its regeneration, and leaving only footsteps in our wake. We should be working symbiotically with the earth as well as supporting those strong community bonds that keep local food initiatives moving forward year after year.

Regenerative Ecosystems Arm

Having watched and participated in the" local food movement" for decades, I've seen a consistent community crossover between people who support local food and people who are concerned about our ecosystems. These concerns seem to go hand in hand. An article written in February of 2020 from the Environmental Protection Online[21], states that the five greatest environmental concerns are 1) Deforestation 2) Air Pollution 3) Global Warming, 4) Water Pollution, and 5) Natural Resource Depletion. Agriculture is perhaps the only industry that influences all five of these concerns on a global level. Basically, how we manage our agricultural land influences everyone on the planet. The two cannot be separated.

Moving forward, the gold standard for agriculture needs to be "regenerative organic." The distinction of just organic vs. regenerative organic is important because the organic standard isn't enough. While the National Organic Standard Board (NOSB) champions the job of defining and maintaining "organic" and is highlighted as one of the third party reviewers that helps us to hone in on the quality of our food, their standards don't aspire to regenerate the land. If the approach to farming is regenerative, the following hallmarks would be noted according to Regeneration International[22]:

1. contribute to generating/building soils and soil fertility and health;

2. increase water percolation, water retention, and clean and safe water runoff;

3. increase biodiversity and ecosystem health and resiliency; and

---

[21] Environmental Protection, 5 Biggest Environmental Issues Affecting the US, By Jenna Tsui, Feb 24, 2020. https://eponline.com/articles/2020/02/24/five-biggest-environmental-issues-affecting-the-us.aspx

[22] Regenerative International Website. https://regenerationinternational.org/2017/02/24/what-is-regenerative-agriculture/:

4. invert the carbon emissions of our current agriculture to one of remarkably significant carbon sequestration thereby cleansing the atmosphere of legacy levels of CO_2.

To the average eater, this may seem like a foreign language, but the important thing is to recognize its importance and to choose a farmer who understands its importance or who is choosing a path toward regenerative agriculture. These folks will be able to have conversations about how they're managing their farm, why they're choosing not to use pesticides, how they're managing cover crop rotations, multispecies intensive grazing rotations with farm animals, composting, and water management. Regenerative organic certifications for farms were available for qualifying farms for the first time in 2020. These certifications can help provide a level of transparency that we don't see in many places in our food supply.

The same practices that contribute to generating soil and increased water retention also help to ensure, on some level, that pesticides and additional fertilizers won't be needed. This is important because we all live downstream. If we remember that every time it rains really hard the water runoff needs to go somewhere, then it brings a whole new light to land management. On the farm, which is one of the greatest contributors to water quality, water is life. Without sunlight, high quality soil, and water, plants and animals don't grow well. The plan is to actively maintain soil so that it retains more water. There's then less runoff and more water available for the plants and animals on the farm as well as having less impact on who is affected downstream.

Recently, I had an opportunity to sit down with the Executive Director of the Watershed Committee of the Ozarks (WCO), Mike Kromrey. WCO is a local nonprofit that has been in existence since 1984 whose outreach efforts impact the quality of water in the Springfield, Missouri city public water supply. Our visit was enlightening to say the least. From his perspective, maintaining water quality is entering an exciting new frontier as regulatory agencies are beginning to embrace more holistic solutions. With the consent of the Missouri Department of Natural Resources (MDNR) and the EPA, the City of Springfield hired an engineering firm to assess the Sustainable Return on Investment (SROI) for different interventions to improve water quality and meet regulatory requirements. SROI quantifies the social, economic, and environmental impact of an intervention over a lifetime of the implemented solution, not just the economics of a situation. Low and behold, what this firm told them was that the programs that influence agricultural land management, such as riparian restoration (actively managing the 500ft to the river bank), livestock rotational grazing (moving livestock from one pasture to the next in a rotation sometimes in coordination with other species of animals until it has been entirely grazed), alternative livestock watering systems (provide alternatives to lakes and streams) and public education all have a high SROI with benefit to cost ratios from two to three to one. Had the consideration simply been for direct outcome relative to cost, these solutions may not have been as appealing.

Ultimately, the greatest limitation over the years to moving these efforts forward has been that of funding. WCO has already established programs for riparian restoration, livestock rotational grazing, alternative watering systems, and public education. Maintaining the efforts over time cost money, however. Several years ago, through relationships that WCO had with City Utilities, Springfield's Utility Company, they had the opportunity to lease some unused farmland to the south of Fellows Lake, Springfield's city water supply. WCO helped improve the rotational grazing system and subleased the property to a local producer with the understanding that the land be managed regeneratively.

Kromrey is quick to point out that everyone wins in this sort of situation. The farmer has access to property at a fair price, spends less time and money feeding his cattle hay in the winter, the microbiota of the soil is maintained, the soil builds back over time because the water is retained on the property more significantly and the cows are happier because they have more robust forage for a longer growing season. The water that does run off below the property that enters the lake carries fewer nutrients and bacteria, so the water remains higher quality and the fish don't suffer because the additional nutrients that facilitate algae bloom don't exist. Sounds like the epitome of the perfect symbiotic relationship between people, the animals, and the land. It also sounds so simple, but this needs to be taught to farmers again because many have bought into the conventional agricultural understanding that it can't be done without large machinery and significant other agricultural inputs.

WCO and Mike Kromrey's efforts have not gone unnoticed. Last year, they were awarded $3.1 million to continue their efforts with local producers. Grant applications submitted in cooperation with other governmental and nongovernmental entities as well as James River Basin Partnership, another water quality nonprofit, received $2.1 million from NRCS "to implement systems that conserve water and soil resources, improve the health of wildlife habitats and increase climate resilience." Perhaps the most novel part of their plan is the Buy Protect Sell approach to land management. This allows the landowner to apply for federal funds for a portion of the purchased land with the understanding that there will be an agricultural easement on the property that dictates that the land will need to be managed regeneratively. This means that over the long term the land will be protected and used in a manner that supports the land, the farm animals, the people, and the environment.

> "Conservation is getting nowhere because it is incompatible with our Abrahamic concept of land. We abuse land because we regard it as a commodity belonging to us. When we see land as a community to which we belong, we may begin to use it with love and respect." —Aldo Leopold

Remember, we all live downstream. The idea that we have to manage our farmland well in order to maintain water quality isn't new but has fallen out of favor because of the enormity of the presence of large-scale conventional agriculture in our country. Our water quality directly impacts our aquatic life. Aquatic life is also impacted by the more toxic pesticide residues and other toxic compounds washed downstream. This is concerning because the increased concentration within this aquatic life (bioaccumulation) and subsequent increase within the food chain (biomagnification) not only impacts aquatic life itself but also the end consumption is oftentimes accomplished by us humans. Studies are mostly done on individual species of aquatic life, which limits the understanding of potential for what's known as the "overall total body burden" for those of us trying to eat "healthier" by including more fish in our diets, meaning more fish may actually expose us to much more toxic chemicals.

The EPA distinguishes between point and nonpoint source contaminants to our water supply. Point source is a single identifiable source. Nonpoint source comes from places like land runoff, precipitation, bacteria from livestock, excessive fertilizer, pesticides, and sediments from improperly managed construction, crop, and forest lands with no specific identifiable source. "States report the nonpoint source is the leading remaining cause of water quality problems." according to the EPA[23], but we have no safeguards in place to ensure that land is managed in a fashion that supports water quality. The challenge here is that agricultural runoff occurs everywhere because our industrialized systems add nitrogen, phosphorus, and potassium back into the soil as well as other inorganic amendments. In doing so without "fixing" it in place, like a regenerative system would approach, it's headed downstream or into the air.

A recent point source example includes one done on PFAS or polyfluoroalkyl substances, found present throughout the Yadkin-Pee Dee river foods chain in North and South Carolina.[24] In this study done by North Carolina University, there were no known plausible industrial inputs in the region. These tests were done across the food chain, so it included larger fish all the way down to the biofilm or the stuff that accumulates on boats when placed in the water. Insects that eat the biofilm were the highest. PFAS are found in food packaging, nonstick pans, wiring, cleaning supplies, paints, paper and many other common household items. PFAS are a health concern because of their associations with testicular cancer, kidney cancer, and endocrine disruption in human beings. For

---

[23] EPA website. https://www.epa.gov/nps/ basic-information-about-nonpoint-source-nps-pollution

[24] PFAS in North Carolina Rivers, North Carolina University, June 5, 2020. https:// www.sciencedaily.com/releases/2020/06/200605165909.htm

reference, PFAS are called forever chemicals because they do not break down readily in nature.

The EPA even had a work group publication on the PFAS contaminants in the river back in November of 2020. Their one recommendation was to include permit requirements for phased-in monitoring and best management practices, as appropriate, taking into consideration when PFAS are expected to be present in point source wastewater discharges.[25] Again, the problem here is that the study listed above clearly states that there's no point source or any single industry obviously responsible for the contamination. A study done in April 2021 by *The Guardian* in cooperation with *Consumer Reports* (CR) indicates that 118 out of 120 sample sites or public water supplies across the country have PFAS or a derivative above the limit set by CR scientists.[26] The EPA has finally set the legally enforceable upper limit for PFAS. The current unenforceable limit is 70 parts per trillion for PFAS and its byproducts. The EPA plans to establish a standard by 2023 and a proposed roadmap to address both the environmental and human impacts through 2024.

In a sustainable regenerative ecosystem, these sorts of concerns would need to be addressed quite directly. A consumer interested in being part of the solution has their hands tied because no one is sure where the offending substance came from, unlike the agricultural amendments that disrupt the soil and allow for all of these "chemicals" to go downstream that has a generally identifiable source. Remembering that the soil is life, meaning that the biology in soil is what aids in retaining water where it falls, is central to the health of our climate and is quite an important concept. Compacted dirt from tractors running all over

---

[25] EPA website, Risk Management for Per- and Polyfluoroalkyl Substances (PFAS) under TSCA, January 2023. https://www.sciencedirect.com/science/article/pii/S0160412019307160?via%3Dihub

[26] Consumer Reports, How Safe Is Our Drinking Water? By Ryan Felton, with additional reporting from Lisa Gill of *Consumer Reports* and Lewis Kendall for *The Guardian*. March 31, 2021 https://www.consumerreports.org/water-quality/how-safe-is-our-drinking-water-a0101771201/

the ground like industrialized agriculture supports doesn't retain water very well. Neither does dirt left behind from clear cutting a forest and burning the leftovers leaving the earth to recover on its own. And concrete retains water even more poorly than either of the first three examples. With farmland being bought up at an enormous rate and being turned into strip malls and residential areas, the result is that the water that falls ends up going somewhere else and the temperature rises in these places as does the water running off of them. Mother Nature's ability to mitigate the damage from this is limited without her greatest earthly resource, the soil, intact.

Regeneratively managed soil purposefully retains the good biology in the soil and basically lets mother nature do her thing. I recently took Soil Food Web courses from Dr Elaine Ingham to learn more about soil biology and to pull together the soil, water, and health connection. My understanding about what she presents in class is that healthy soil will retain water longer, so it requires less watering, and it provides increased yields with fewer to no agricultural inputs. How is this possible? The plants send out exudates that attract bacteria and fungi in the soil and, when nurtured, build microaggregates or soil structure that helps retain water. Soil bacteria produce glues that hold these aggregates together. Additionally, the bacteria and fungi attract predators, such as protozoa as well as nematodes and microarthropods that then feed off of them. They then excrete waste or digested bacteria and fungi back into the soil that then makes the "waste" plant available for growth. These larger predators then help to form macroaggregates in the soil that allow the soil to retain even more water. As the soil aggregates and fungi grow, so does the retention of carbon into the soil structure. Ideally, the encouragement of the soil would be toward a higher fungal structure, as this portion of the biology retains more carbon, but large amounts isn't necessarily ideal for all plants. Regardless, a lack of adequate biology is usually the greatest concern in most horticultural situations. As long as the soil has adequate ground cover and organic matter, the biome does quite well. While this seems so simple, our largest food system on the planet doesn't allow for mother nature to function at her best. As previously mentioned, this also diminishes the nutritional quality of the end plant product as well.

Interestingly, when looking at surface water runoff, it's an easy extension to look at the agriculture that contributes to significant detrimental runoff and CO_2 emissions. While the point source example above is most likely an unidentified industrial dumping, the way we do agriculture significantly impacts whether carbon is sequestered into the soil or whether it's blown off as CO_2 into the air. Same with nitrogen, although the term used for nitrogen is fixing. It's either fixed or not fixed, and this determines whether it goes downstream, stays present in the soil or up into the air. Simply put, most of our agricultural land is managed conventionally with large amounts of inorganic amendments, heavy tilling, pesticides, herbicides, fungicides, or insecticides year after year to attempt to support the growth of the plants. When managed this way, the portion of the soil that helps to retain phosphorus, sequester CO_2, and fix nitrogen, the biology in the soil, becomes limited and often killed by these amendments and processes surrounding it. The only way to nurture the biology in the soil is to add back, support, and feed the biology what it needs to survive. What we do with conventional agriculture is the equivalent of putting a human being on antibiotics and Tums chronically for an entire lifetime and expecting it to feel better without changing diet or exercising. The problem is that the root cause of the problem is never addressed. In other words, we need to discontinue our industrialized model, so biology can survive.

The industrialization of food in America supports subsidization, mechanization, fertilization, and genetic modification of our food. Our capitalistic American ideals have become too focused on bottom-line dollar-driven policy that has essentially put the vibrant farmer out of business. But this rejuvenation of the small, regenerative farm is, in fact, what needs to happen to influence these issues. The larger the farm, the more likely to require increased mechanization and the compaction that follows. Small Vibrant farms have the ability to not only become their own ecosystems but also viable contributors to a local food economy. The next arm of the compass explores how we can not only support our local regenerative farmers and our ecosystems but also our local food economy.

Thriving Local Economies Arm

The fastest growing segments of the food industry are local, sustainable organic foods.[27] Organic Trade Association's (OTA) latest Organic Industry Survey shows between 2020 and 2021, organic sales surpassed $63 billion, with $1.4 billion (2%) total growth over the year.[28] People are wanting to connect more with their food, and their food needs to be grown with a purpose to improve environmental and personal health as well as support animal welfare. They want to know more about how their food is raised and grown, desire food transparency, and are willing to spend a little more for it. This growth has been driven by increasing health concerns and the understanding that our food can be our medicine or our poison.

In order for the Vibrant farm to be the center point of a local economy, there must be a strong community. Community ties and building relationships allow for the economic success of a local food community. Think about the economic impact if every time we, as consumers of goods, purposefully chose a local product instead of going to Walmart or Amazon to purchase a product. Yes, it can be a little more work but when done with purpose, the result is that a larger percentage of the hard-earned dollars of the consumers stays local.

[27] Global News Wire, Demand for Local and Organic Food Is on the Rise, Positively Impacting the Food and Beverage Market, as per the Global Food And Beverage Market Report 2020, October 15, 2020 The Business Research Company. https://www.globenewswire.com/news-release/2020/10/15/2109006/0/en/Demand-For-Local-And-Organic-Food-Is-On-The-Rise-Positively-Impacting-The-Food-And-Beverage-Market-As-Per-The-Global-Food-And-Beverage-Market-Report-2020.html

[28] Organic Trade Association Website, 2019 organic sales Organic Industry Survey, U.S. Organic Industry Survey 2022 https://ota.com/organic-market-overview/organic-industry-survey

An IMPLAN (Impact Analysis for Planning) study done in Central Oregon in October of 2017 by OSU[29]" showed that producers created a total of 28 full and part-time jobs and generated $1.5 million in sales, with $248,000 in wages and salaries on their farm operations." And "Unlike imported foods, which retain $0.28 for every dollar spent, 76% of sales by local producers stayed in the local economy. This means that the money spent by producers on their supplies, such as seeds and gas, created an additional 11 jobs and $1.1 million in additional sales throughout the region's economy." The action that supports this is that a local producer as opposed to a commodity producer is more likely to look for supplies locally. This helps to support additional jobs locally as well. The additional sacrifice from the consumer involves some additional time spent researching where a product can be obtained locally as well as, perhaps, some planning if not available year-round or if in low supply. We, the American consumers, would have to give up some of our convenience to support our local farmers.

This decentralized agriculture supports local food economies, however. Decentralized agriculture means that the larger more "centralized" supply chains are broken down into smaller more locally distributed chains that are more resilient when a small part of it breaks down. Think of the map of the United States with five spider webs in it that don't overlap much. This is the larger centralized food system. Now with the same space of the United States that you envisioned the larger web in, put thousands of small ones, some larger than others but all also interconnect on some level. In the center of each one, there's a vibrant farm. This is what it used to look like all over rural America. When one supply chain went down, there were others close by. Local businesses thrived because they were supported locally. I will discuss more about centralized agriculture in Chapter 5.

This decentralization is significant because it has the ability, if organized with the purpose of supporting local entrepreneurs rather than an industrialized

---

[29] Economic Impact of Local Food Producers in Central Oregon: A Survey Based IMPLAN Model Incorporating the USDA AMS Toolkit Guidelines, October 2017 https://agsci.oregonstate.edu/sites/agscid7/files/economicimpact_localfoods_centraloregon.pdf

system, to help buffer these businesses against the lack of enforcement with anti-trust laws as well. Remember, a large number of local producers have been put out of business because of the lack of enforcement of these laws as well as an ever-encroaching decrease in the monies that the local producer actually takes home because of the way it's set up.

I recently had an opportunity to talk with Mike Callicrate, owner of Callicrate Cattle Company and Ranch Foods Direct. Mike lamented as our conversation started that he is one of a very few independent cattlemen left in Colorado. Slowly, over time, many abandoned cattle farming because it's no longer profitable. Mike has spent his fair share of time in litigation and attempting legislation around changing the system but to no avail. He's been able to weather the storm from the industry because, some time ago, he switched his business model to take out the middleman, which historically takes a large percentage of the cut, by doing his own processing and selling directly to the consumer. "This means that a substantially greater amount of money goes back directly to the producer even after processing fees and everyone is paid, as it bypasses the big meat packer, retailer, and food service industries that take the largest percentage of the cut. This number can be an astounding 75 to 80% back to the producer versus 33%, currently USDA uses 44% for farm share numbers. This is the difference between staying in business and not for a rancher. Basically, the producer has lost around half of their share of the consumer beef dollar to middlemen."

This model also includes a better paid and a more skilled local workforce which puts the money back into the local economy rather than into the pockets of the propped up and, some would argue, corrupt industrialized system. Coupling this model in 2017 with The Peak to Plains Food Hub also provided an opportunity to support additional local businesses that were like minded about supply chains, keeping them as local as possible, given the limitations of the system. During COVID, Peak to Plains continued to run a virtual food hub with drive-through, curbside pick-up one day a week. Some of the partners in the food hub included a brewer, gourmet meat pie company, baker, distillery, food truck, local farm, as well as additional aggregation for other food hubs.

Food hubs are a great example of how some communities are gathering food supply chains to a single location and providing wholesale market access. As with Peak to Plains, food hubs across the country are central gathering places within a region to aggregate, process, store, and market local food products. Some also offer technical support and training for local farmers, veterans or folks with a history of incarceration who are trying to learn new skills. Yet, others function in cooperation with retail operations or large institutions to become that ever so important anchor or pull through for end product retail use. Some even offer their own value-added food products, which provides a whole new functionality beyond just distribution of food. Mid-America Food Hub, LLC is one such food hub in Pilot Grove Missouri. Mid-America offers over 40 different fruits and vegetables as well as value-added products and meats. There are hundreds of food hubs across the country now, https://www.ams.usda.gov/local-food-directories/foodhubs. This is a link to all registered food hubs across the county. If one goes to this site, it appears that there's quite a bit moving on the local food front, and there certainly has been expansion. But is it enough? Folks who do this sort of work believe there needs to be dozens of vibrant farms and at least one food hub in every 10-15 county region, but we aren't even close to meeting this mark.

Memberships in food hubs, while having access to aggregation opportunities, unfortunately don't provide ownership of the entity itself. In some communities, we build our lives around well-manicured golf courses. Why not local food? Something that nurtures the health of our communities in quite a different way. Mike Callicrate is proposing a development around the ownership of a cooperative entity, much like a food hub, except individual businesses have an actual ownership of the entity itself as well as a storefront location. The proposed Pikes Marketplace Cooperative is a cooperative of local businesses that would become a destination for community members to shop where transparency of food product and wares are tantamount to the sale of the item itself, business are owner-operated, and additional ancillary businesses are created as extensions of the support of local food and local businesses. For example, a grain mill would be an important additional business to support the brewery, the distillery, as well as the bread baker. There's still shared storage and refrigeration but also opportunities as a gathering place that helps to support the community that will come together in cooperation with such a venture. Sounds a bit like the fictitious community in this book called Vitality where everyone thrives, but this is the direction that we need to start thinking and organizing in order to truly economically support local food systems that can buffer our communities from the industrialized system.

Where Do At-Risk Populations Fit in?

There's increasing emphasis on food insecurity and what it means to individual communities. What if there were a gradual change over the subsidizing of community food rather than the commodity food talked about in Chapter 1? If community food were taken to a larger scale, we could, as Dr. John Ikerd, an agricultural economist and professor emeritus of the University of Missouri-Columbia promotes, develop Community Food Utilities (CFU)[30] . These utilities would be based upon the identified needs of each individual community around a city or region. Each region could be responsible for providing a food system evaluation indicating the strengths and weaknesses of their local food system. Funding could then be provided relative to Asset Based Community Development (ABCD) for each region to ensure the success of these endeavors. The assets of each organization or individual with skin in the game, so to speak, would be considered working forward. Clear rules of engagement and boundaries would be established within these communities to ensure that these common resources were managed effectively. This would, in fact, impact the issue of hunger more than a commodity program because each community would accept responsibility to ensure that no one went hungry, with an emphasis on healthy, fresh, local food.

Dr Ikerd believes that discretionary hunger is a market failure and will continue to exist until local communities have the ability to interfere with the

---

[30] Ikerd, J. White Paper on Community Food Utilities. https://sites.google.com/site/communityfoodutility/enough-good-food-for-all-a-community-food-utility

current industrialized food system that promotes and supports junk food in low-income communities. Discretionary hunger, in this case, means that hunger is at the discretion of the system rather than the interpersonal community relationships. To change this would require a level of understanding from the average consumer about local and regional food systems and the desire of local businesses and consumers to invest in the community in a very different way.

This part of the paradigm shift insists that instead of supporting the local food bank, which tends to be the endpoint for a lot of nonperishable foods from the industrialized system, there should be allocation of some funding and cooperation around putting some farmland into food production or ensuring that everyone has enough access to healthy foods and/or an opportunity to help produce it. Teaching a person to fish rather than providing the fish to eat makes some good sense if we want a productive society. When I asked Mike if this would be considered as a part of the Pikes Marketplace Cooperative, he didn't hesitate when answering that it would have to be. True community considers all of its citizens, not just those who can afford to start businesses. If all citizens are taken care of, everyone benefits in some form or another.

Think of the local farmers during the COVID-19 crisis who didn't increase their prices because they knew that people were out of work and couldn't afford a $20 pork chop. It was more important to maintain the relationship over profits because, eventually, COVID wasn't going to be an issue anymore. This is the epitome of how the local food system is more resilient. Think of the strong ties in your own community that build financial opportunities separate from food. The question then becomes, how can we support these relationships to ensure that the community continues to invest in local food systems? In a capitalistic society, grass roots that help to address and solve major food systems mismanagement can still make a difference, especially when everyone wins and the community sees value in this, whether it's reduced crime rates or just a desire to see all humanely treated and fed.

In Southwest Missouri, there are some fantastic local examples of these sorts of relationships between water quality nonprofits, business entities that integrate with nonprofit organizations as well as additional public/private relationships. This sort of relationship building isn't limited to rural America. Urban farming relationships also exist that support local food endeavors as well. Perhaps my favorite example is the 2,658-square-foot garden on the rooftop of Boston Medical Center that helps to feed at-risk populations. According to a 2019 article in *Reuters*,[31] physicians can actually prescribe more vegetables to the hospital's patients because most of its produce goes to the hospital-based food pantry. It also saved the hospital approximately $10,000 in food costs for one year. There's really no downside to these sorts of efforts.

Change Needs to be Not Just Well Intentioned but Well Thought Out

There was a recent and profound example of well-intentioned agricultural policy change in Sri Lanka that went awry. The policy was meant to address health concerns, specifically, chronic kidney failure that appears to affect farmers in dry regions of Sri Lanka disproportionately. This kidney failure has been attributed to their agricultural practices. In response, the president of Sri Lanka in May of 2021 mandated an immediate policy change for the country to change agricultural practices to go all organic with no synthetic fertilizers or pesticides. To be clear, most of their agricultural practices are dependent upon these inputs. The impact of this in the midst of some other economic issues has led to some rioting in the streets and large-scale hunger amongst its people.

This country by some economic standards would have been considered previously self-sufficient regarding food, now finds itself importing one of its main dietary staples, rice. These sorts of scenarios don't happen overnight but are coupled with some extreme circumstances internationally and poor policy decisions over the last several years. The country had some losses of income from

---

[31] Mathias, T. A Boston Hospital with A farm on Its Roof Seeks to Inspire Others, July 25, 2019. https://www.reuters.com/article/us-health-hospital-farming/a-boston-hospital-with-a-farm-on-its-roof-seeks-to-inspire-others-idUSKCN1UK29P

tourism due to COVID, extreme spending on infrastructure in the last decade that didn't generate income, a populist tax cut decreasing income to the new government, further exacerbating the debt-to-income ratio for the country. This all occurred prior to the implementation of agricultural policy attempting to support the health of the 2 million farmers that make up 30% of the country's workforce. The country has now also defaulted on debts in the midst of extreme inflation, gas shortages, and rolling blackouts to conserve energy. In summary, some well-intentioned but poorly thought out and unsupported policy decisions exacerbated an already challenging situation. Policy that expects an overnight change for systems that take years to change even when approached with a purpose, much less for a group of farmers who didn't have the skills to accomplish the policy, was destined for failure from the start.

Because this is a book about agriculture and health, let's first discuss what may be influencing kidney failure as well as the economic burden of kidney failure on a third world country that has a predominantly agriculturally based economy, ill-equipped to handle the increasing volume of these patients. Medical science has not fully determined the direct cause of the chronic kidney failure (CKDu) of unknown origin in Sri Lanka that started in the 1990s. Initially it was occurring within certain villages and families but now appears to no longer be limiting itself to the dry regions of the country. For the record, kidneys function quite poorly when dehydrated, which may be one of the causative factors. Ninety-five percent of CKD around the world can be attributed to high blood pressure or diabetes, and that's why this CKDu is special. These folks aren't overweight or struggling with high blood pressure. Statistically, however, the numbers are rising on the whole, which led to the policy change surrounding agricultural inputs. Sri Lanka uses a subsidy program for inorganic fertilizers, which encouraged their use, until their ban in May of 2021. The ban, now lifted because of the crisis, has not allowed for an increase in their use because of worldwide shortages. In Sri Lanka, whether perceived or real, there's a general understanding that pesticides will help to increase yields, regardless of environmental or human health impact. This has led to a significant increase in use of pesticides.

In Chapter 6, there's much more exploration of agricultural practices and their influence on our health. The current running theories regarding CKDu in Sri Lanka according in the literature include cadmium (a very nephrotoxic heavy metal) from phosphate fertilizers; arsenic, which is sequestered by rice; lead, a toxic heavy metal; nitrates, also found in fertilizers; home brews, which are notorious for toxins and heavy metals; mycotoxins in grains; and fluoride from pesticide residues as well as a high concentration in soil and groundwater already and, subsequently, in food. Eighty percent of the population relies on groundwater for their hydration needs; therefore, anything that influences the quality of the groundwater also influences the health of the largest part of the population. CKD rates are higher in certain farming villages and start affecting them at a young age as evidenced by biochemical markers that show up quite early in life before overt symptoms of kidney failure occur. Its influence has expanded from initially some agricultural villages to potentially impacting parts of the entire county. The cause is most likely multifactorial in nature rather than one simple cause in a third world country that has a high degree of malnutrition and is not equipped to handle a problem of this magnitude.

One article by Sunil J. Wimalawansa, entitled "Public Health Interventions for Chronic Diseases: Cost–Benefit Modelizations for Eradicating Chronic Kidney Disease of Multifactorial origin (CKDmfo/ CKDu) From Tropical Countries"[32], addresses the issue from the preventative side. While the article addresses a multifactorial approach, the benefits of providing clean drinking water alone "while costing $0.67 million/year, is expected to reduce healthcare and the associated costs by more than $15.6 million (1.8 billion Sri Lankan rupees) per year, even without including the opportunity cost…. A 24-fold cost-to-benefit ratio." Why not try?

---

[32] Sunil J. Wimalawansa, Public Health Interventions for Chronic Diseases: Cost–Benefit Modelizations for Eradicating Chronic Kidney Disease of Multifactorial Origin (CKDmfo/ CKDu) from Tropical Countries, *Heliyon*, Volume 5, Issue 10, 2019. https://www.sciencedirect.com/science/article/pii/S2405844019359699#:~:text=In%20Sri%20Lanka%2C%20the%20governmental,this%20is%20a%20recurring%20cost.

Just because this particular policy change wasn't successful doesn't mean that it wasn't a good idea. However, the overall message here needs to be that we shouldn't throw the baby out with the bathwater. While the policy change here was well-intentioned, without some additional support for farmers to learn how to farm organically or regeneratively, the whole system collapsed. It's not possible to make this change overnight. A step-wise phase-in makes the most sense as well as incorporating some incentivization or subsidization for those who choose an agricultural path that supports the health of its citizens. The same would have to occur in this country in order to encourage a safe and effective switch over to agricultural standards that support the health of our citizens, our communities, and our environment.

The greatest problem is, in fact, that there isn't enough local food available to meet demand, and there are limited networks to support the demand that does exist. We need to grow more real food and set up the supply chains that support our local economies. Communities build lives together. Industry just builds wealth. Generally speaking, the pockets of local entrepreneurs don't get rich when it comes to food systems. The agricultural giants become more and more wealthy because of the subsidies.

Calibration of the Compass

It's all about prioritization. According to the website Modern Farmer, 41% of the agricultural land sold goes to development of rural areas and 175 acres of farmland is lost every hour or about 3 acres every minute.[33] Every time farmland is sold to a developer, we lose some more of our precious vibrant farm community opportunities. The challenge is that a developer will most likely pay more than another farmer for the land. It's not a stretch to see how enticing this is when headed toward retirement. Without some dedication to maintaining the land in a farming capacity, many of the farms previously in production will be turned

---

[33] Modern Farmer Website. https://modernfarmer.com/2018/05/10-numbers-that-show-how-much-farmland-were-losing-to-development/

into strip malls and contribute to the concrete jungle or urban development. This is perhaps our biggest issue when it comes to the overall food production. We're losing our farms.

Farmland trusts such as American Farmland Trust https://farmland.org/about/ protect farmland so that when donated, it will only go back to farms and, in some cases, regenerative farming.

So, from the Vibrant farms and local food systems perspective, if we take care of the earth through our farming practices, not only will this farm provide us with healthier food options but it can also provide significant anchoring to a local food economy as well as value to our communities and ecosystems. Remember, all health is local. This concept cannot be emphasized enough. If our built, social, economic, and natural environments are healthy, so will our people be healthy. There's a symbiotic relationship between the earth and our bodies that, once aware of, should be embraced as one of the most important opportunities on the planet rather than something to be limited by. Our current system doesn't allow for this. It can't. It's not put together in a fashion that allows for the average consumer to understand what they're eating and where it's coming from, much less have a relationship with the person providing the food product unless, of course, it's yourself. It keeps us separate from understanding what's going into our bodies and how it affects the earth.

So, if we, as consumers, shift our focus to food consumption with a purpose, it sheds a whole new light on the act of eating. If the interrelationship between real food raised regeneratively and the health of our people, our planet, our community relationships, and our economy were understood and presented as of vital importance, the industrialized system would have less of a stronghold on our health and our livelihoods. This, in fact, is the calibration or shift of the paradigm that's needed in order to improve our health and help the earth support her own ability to heal herself as well. Let's now try to understand more about what's known in order to ask the right questions to encourage this paradigm shift forward.

4.
Blind Leading the Blind

A friend texted me a few weeks ago. Her text indicated that her child was vomiting again. It happens quite a bit, but it wasn't until the last few weeks that she began to realize that it was associated with a pasta product she had been feeding her. I asked her to send me a picture of the food product front and back. The back indicated that it basically had one food ingredient, Durum Wheat Semolina, but it was enriched with ferrous sulfate (iron) and some B vitamins, including niacin, thiamin mononitrate, riboflavin, and folic acid. Not too complicated or concerning for a food label. It also had the usual promotions of contents it never contained: 0 Saturated Fat, 0 Sodium, Cholesterol Free. It was produced in Italy. So, I asked if she ate other pasta or wheat products without any vomiting or other side effects and she said yes. I let her know that some food products have undeclared ingredients as well as potential contaminants to which she could possibly be reacting. The recommendation I gave her was to stay away from the brand. The question remains, however, what was causing her vomiting?

This story isn't unusual in my practice. And anyone who has to actively manage a chronic health condition that requires knowing what's in the food supply will tell you how challenging it is. Some folks take it to the extreme of sending the food product off to a lab and have the food product tested to attempt to pin down the culprit within the food. Even this approach has some limitations, as it can be like looking for a needle in a haystack. My greatest concern, as a nutritional health practitioner, is the challenge people face when they really do want to take charge of their health. How do we know what we're eating if there are additives or ingredients in our foods that we don't know about? And what's allowed in our food supply that's not necessarily supporting our health? From the labeling laws in America, there really is very limited food transparency in America and very limited enforcement of what's considered the law.

What's Food Transparency?

Food transparency can quite simply be defined as being allowed to know everything you need to know about the food you're eating in order to be able to make an informed decision about your food choices. Where do the ingredients come from? How are they packaged? How is it processed? And who is producing the food? Food transparency, despite its limited availability, in America is one of the hottest trends in the food industry because consumers are demanding to know more about their food. This can allow for opportunities to eat healthier when food manufacturers are providing more information about their products, therefore, allowing for more informed food choices. Unfortunately, many food labels make statements as a marketing tool rather than a point of transparency. We consumers must continue to remain diligent with reading food and ingredient labels and continue to ask questions in an effort to remain informed about what we're putting into our bodies.

Some food companies claim to provide full food transparency. Be sure to read all the small details with these companies and/or make a phone call to them to ask more questions if this is part of their promotion. The word "transparency" as with any wording on a food label is at risk of being utilized as a buzz term. There's no official meaning; therefore, the term could mean whatever the manufacturer wants it to mean. Regardless, full transparency would be great because the consumer isn't left out of knowing what's being eaten. Sadly, most never come any closer to food transparency than the listing of ingredients, potential allergens, a breakdown of select macro and micronutrients and the percentage of Daily Reference Intakes (DRI) that they're obligated to provide. The rules surrounding food labels are pretty loose to begin with, much less informative about what we're eating. The following was pulled straight from the FDA website showing the contradiction from the first sentence to the last regarding requirements for labels.

"Food manufacturers are required to list all ingredients in the food on the label. On a product label, the ingredients are listed in order of predominance, with the ingredients used in the greatest amount first, followed in descending order by those in smaller amounts. The label must list the names of any FDA-certified color additives (e.g., FD&C Blue No. 1 or the abbreviated name, Blue 1). But some ingredients can be listed collectively as "flavors," "spices," "artificial flavoring," or in the case of color additives exempt from certification, "artificial colors," without naming each one. Declaration of an allergenic ingredient in a collective or single color, flavor, or spice could be accomplished by simply naming the allergenic ingredient in the ingredient list."[34]

If a manufacturer is able to "collectively" list ingredients, it would be impossible for a consumer to know what they're reacting to if a reaction occurs. This is one of the many reasons why I recommend avoiding processed foods entirely. There's no way to know what we're really eating, and the awareness that food sensitivities play a role in our overall health is rising. So, while we generally know what's in our food, we really don't know enough to make an educated decision. We can't. Recently, I had a patient in the hospital who had a corn allergy and as I was reading some labels of the individual products on our shelves at the hospital, I noticed that our flavored soy milk had "natural flavorings" in it. I called the manufacturer directly and, sure enough, the "natural flavorings" included corn. It wasn't listed as an ingredient on the food label because it's not one of the most frequent food allergens but quite common in our food supply.

In America, the FDA is also in charge of policing ingredients in food products via a designation known as GRAS food ingredients. Here is an excerpt from the FDA website regarding what this means.

---

[34] FDA Website, Overview of Food Ingredients, Additives and Colors Revised April 2010. https://www.fda.gov/food/food-ingredients-packaging/overview-food-ingredients-additives-colors#qalabel

"GRAS" is an acronym for the phrase **G**enerally **R**ecognized **A**s **S**afe. Under sections 201(s) and 409 of the Federal Food, Drug, and Cosmetic Act (the Act), any substance that is intentionally added to food is a food additive, that is subject to premarket review and approval by FDA, unless the substance is generally recognized, among qualified experts, as having been adequately shown to be safe under the conditions of its intended use, or unless the use of the substance is otherwise excepted from the definition of a food additive.

So, as part of a regulatory review of food products, any food additive that has been allowed on the shelves of the grocery store should be considered safe for us to eat. The problem with this, is that, in America, we eat too many processed foods, and there are concerns now being explored that the "collective" of all these additives, while considered in the overall potential exposure, may quite simply be too much for our body systems to manage. While GRAS additives are proposed to be an overestimate of exposures, there is evidence that food additives can disrupt the microbiome and create an inflammatory response. Some additives have even been pulled from the market. Most recently non-natural-occurring trans fats or partially hydrogenated oils (PHOs) fall in that category. In June 2015, the FDA allowed for a three-year phase out of trans fats due to the possible hardship to the soybean growers as the majority of trans fats were made from soybeans. They would now need to find other end product markets for their soybeans. While sympathetic to the plight of the soybean grower, most soybeans in America are genetically modified, and soy is in a large volume of highly processed products. What about the health of the unaware consumer? Should we not be as concerned about them?

- Officially a food label must contain:
- statement of identity (What's it?)
- the product's net weight,
- manufacturer's address,

- nutrition facts, and

- ingredients list, listed from heaviest to lightest.

The nutrition facts must include:

- serving size,

- nutrients, and

- certain vitamins and minerals expressed as a % of DRI.

This is very little information for the American consumer to work from. The new rules around food labeling and GMO or bioengineered foods should be applicable by the time this book goes to publication. This will include some additional transparency but, according to the new rule, the National Bioengineered Food Disclosure Standard or NBFDS considers only a few foods to be considered bioengineered.[35] These include apples, canola, corn, eggplants, papaya, pineapple, potatoes, salmon, soybean, squash, and sugar beets. The law exempts animal feed, pet foods and personal care products. It also exempts a food if it's listed as the third ingredient (after water, stock or broth) or later or if the food product has undergone some form or processing that keeps genetically modified material from being undetected. Under this premise, canola oil and soda pop would be exempt from having to be labeled despite the number one and perhaps only ingredient being defined as genetically modified or bioengineered. Further, the USDA doesn't plan to do spot checks on food products. Like the supplement industry, investigation will be based on a complaint basis. I see no transparency in this.

---

[35] Guide to U.S. Regulation of Genetically Modified Food and Agricultural Biotechnology Products, Pew Trusts. https://www.pewtrusts.org/~/media/legacy/uploadedfiles/wwwpewtrustsorg/reports/food_and_biotechnology/hhsbiotech-0901pdf.pdf

"Reading Between the Lines" on Labels and Packaging

In 2013, regulations were enacted that required manufacturers to label gluten containing foods and provided the following definition for not being able to label as "gluten free":

- An ingredient that's any type of wheat, rye, barley, or crossbreeds of these grains,

- An ingredient derived from these grains that has *not* been processed to remove gluten, or,

- an ingredient derived from these grains that *has* been processed to remove gluten, but results in the food containing more than 20 ppm of gluten.

Prior to the passage of this law, there had been no definition for "gluten free" with regard to food labeling. This is important because the rates of celiac disease, for which the only treatment is a gluten-free diet, are on the rise with a current incidence of one in 100, as well as an underlying systemic response for a large percentage of the population known as non-celiac gluten sensitivity (NCGS). Folks with NCGS don't necessarily have an allergic reaction to gluten but have a clear set of symptoms similar to irritable bowel syndrome (intermittent gas, bloating, constipation and diarrhea) that resolve when removing gluten from the diet.

Per the Food Allergen Labeling and Consumer Protection Act of 2004 or FALCPA[36], if any of the most common allergens (milk, egg, peanut, tree nuts, soy, wheat, fish, and crustacean shellfish) are present they must be listed. These food allergens account for 90% of all food allergies in America. Certainly, other foods can cause allergies, but because these represent the vast majority, they're specifically represented by FALCPA. The leftover 10% leaves a lot of room for concern with food allergies on the rise with one in 10 adults and one in 13

---

[36] FDA Website. https://www.fda.gov/food/food-allergens-gluten-free-guidance-documents-regulatory-information/food-allergen-labeling-and-consumer-protection-act-2004-falcpa

children with a diagnosed food allergy and 175,000 people per year headed to the ER with anaphylactic, life-threatening reactions.[37]

Additionally, any claims made on the label must be 100% accurate. So, if a claim is made about a food being fat free it needs to not have any fat in it. A food cannot claim to mitigate, prevent, treat or cure any disease. But these limitations are, in fact, not enough because studies show packaging has a strong influence on consumer preference regarding what's purchased. Approximately 80% of snack foods make health claims in their marketing. According to FDA regulations, as long as the food product contains less than 10% saturated fat it can be called low fat. And if a product contains at least 10% of two other nutrients it can be considered a good source of that nutrient. Marketing with words such as "natural" can be confusing, especially if it comes along with marketing earthy colors. The average consumer actually believes that they're eating a healthier food product. The following is a quote from the FDA website:

> The FDA has considered the term "natural" to mean that nothing artificial or synthetic (including all color additives regardless of source) has been included in, or has been added to, a food that would not normally be expected to be in that food. However, this policy was not intended to address food production methods, such as the use of pesticides, nor did it explicitly address food processing or manufacturing methods, such as thermal technologies, pasteurization, or irradiation.[38]

So, this "natural" food product can be grown with pesticides or other agricultural means that don't support either its nutritional content or ecologically sound practices. It doesn't take but a single trip to the health food market, picking

---

[37] FARE Website. https://www.foodallergy.org/resources/facts-and-statistics

[38] FDA website on Use of the Term Natural. https://www.fda.gov/food/food-labeling-nutrition/use-term-natural-food-labeling#:~:text=The%20FDA%20has%20considered%20the,to%20be%20in%20that%20food.

up packages and reading ingredients to understand the depth of the deception, whether intended or not. Food manufacturers are in the business of selling their product and this is BIG money.

So, let's talk about where the rubber meets the road with a real-life example of how a federally subsidized food crop, oats, is labeled and impacts our health in America. My favorite example is with oat cereals. Many make the claim that it's whole grain, may reduce the risk of heart disease, isn't made with genetically modified ingredients, is low fat and a good source of fiber, can help cholesterol, and is an excellent source of iron. All of this is true and not misleading in any way. As you see, there's no specific medical claim with statements prefaced with the words "may reduce" or "can help with," and, by definition, each of their claims can be substantiated. It's no secret that oats are a healthy, high-fiber food choice. A bit misleading to say the least.

Here is what food labels don't tell you.

Every year, the non-GMO crop of oats has glyphosate, one of the most common herbicides in America, sprayed on it. Despite the fact that oats aren't a genetically modified food crop, glyphosate is used as a desiccant to dry the oats out prior to harvest. This practice is common in certain parts of the country, not just for oats but other food crops as well. When the oats are harvested, they have a large dose of glyphosate residue still left on them. When doing the deeper dive into how much residue should be considered the Maximum Residue Limit (MRL), this is where further controversy comes in. There basically is no consensus within the United States or other international agencies on how much is in fact reasonable for human consumption nor is there consistency with regard to testing methods for not only glyphosate but its primary metabolite AMPA. As a consumer, I am somewhat confused about why there is not consensus but I was encouraged to know that it is listed on Prop 65 as a potential carcinogen and that organic products test substantially lower than non organic products for pesticide residues. According to Biodx.co, 33 countries across the world have banned glyphosate from use. Why should we be concerned about eating a large dose of glyphosate? Despite health claims from companies that promote nonorganic oat consumption, the high levels of glyphosate are known endocrine disruptors contributing to oxidative stress of the human body and it's a known cancer-causing agent and a neurotoxin. I'll go into all of this in more depth in Chapter 6.

So here we have a food product that would be considered a healthy gluten-free option that literally may be contributing to the degradation of the health of America because we're generally unaware of how oats are grown in our country. More to the point, we feed it to children who, relative to body size, are receiving a much larger dose per kilogram of body weight than any adult. Concerning to say the least.

Is There a Seal of Approval?

The good news is that there are a variety of third-party reviewers of food products that will place seals of approval on individual products after going through a certification process or that have done their own research and testing. While third-party reviewer systems aren't foolproof, at least, they provide another layer of transparency with regard to our food supply. Some examples of these third-party reviewers are: Certified USDA organic, Certified Humane, NonGMO Project, Certified Naturally Grown, Animal Welfare Approved, American Grassfed Association.

Certified USDA Organic managed by the United States Department of Agriculture relies on inspections of farms to ensure the standards set by the National Organic Standards Board (NOSB) are upheld, https://www.ams.usda.gov/grades-standards/organic-standards/. Foods in this category fall into one of three sub-categories if organically certified.100% organic (100% of ingredients organic), Organic > 70% organic food ingredients, Made with Organic foods < 70% organic food ingredients.

Certified Humane® from Humane Farm Animal Care (HFAC). HFAC operates transparently, publicizing all scientific standards so the public will know exactly how animals protected by their seal of approval are treated. https://certifiedhumane.org/how-we-work/fact-sheet/

The Non-GMO Project North America's only third-party verification and labeling for non-GMO food and products. Visit here https://www.nongmoproject.org/find-non-gmo/verified-products/product-categories/ for a full listing of certified products.

Certified Naturally Grown (CNG) farmers don't use synthetic fertilizers, pesticides, herbicides, or GMOs. Beekeepers employ similar practices on where hives are located. Unlike USDA Certified Organic, CNG is the only certification that relies on peer inspections, transparency, and direct relationships for auditing. For a listing of farmers close to your location visit https://www.certified.naturallygrown.org

Animal Welfare Approved (AWA) is a transparent third party reviewer of animal producers ensuring that animals are raised in their natural environments as well as managed humanely. Visit https://animalwelfareapproved.us/advanced-product-search/ to search for products in your location. AWA also has a grass-fed certification.

American Grassfed Association (AGA) employs a sustainable approach to farm/ranch management designed to enhance land, water, and air quality. AGA uses the standards of animal husbandry in their grazing programs to support humane treatment of welfare of their animals. Search here for producers by state at https://www.americangrassfed.org/producer-profiles/producer-members-by-state/

Regenerative Organic Certification (ROC) promotes soil health, animal welfare, and social fairness. This standard became new in 2020 and certifies farms all over the world. Visit their site at https://regenorganic.org/regenorganic-certified/. This is the standard that I believe holds the most promise for promoting soil regeneration.

While this isn't a comprehensive list, these are some third-party reviewers who encourage transparency as the foundation of their structure as well as practices in food production that encourage a nutritionally healthier end food product. All certifiers have their own seal that can then be displayed proudly on the individual producer's product for marketing purposes. This makes it somewhat easier to choose but, again, doesn't negate the responsibility of the individual consumer to remain diligent by asking questions and reading food labels if available. And here's why. Just because a food product has an organic seal or any third-party seal on it doesn't mean it has been processed into something that's good for you. A good example of this would be crackers at the health food store. Next time you're there, randomly pick up several different boxes and read the label. If there are more than 5 ingredients and you're unsure what they are, perhaps you shouldn't be eating it. As Michael Pollan, a writer for more than 30 years about how we interact with our food and the brokenness of our food systems would say, "Don't eat anything your grandmother wouldn't recognize as food."[39] Sometimes, simple advice brings the point home best. Remember, these additional, nonfood ingredients potentially have a cumulative impact on our microbiome.

Additionally, it needs to be noted that just because there's a third-party reviewer doesn't necessarily ensure you're getting what you think. The organic standard, in particular, has come under the greatest amount of scrutiny for the failures of the USDA to enforce their standard in accordance with the guidelines of the NOSB. An expose published in 2017 by the *Washington Post,* https://www.washingtonpost.com/news/wonk/wp/2017/12/21/organic-food-fraud-leads-congress-to-weigh-bill-doubling-usda-oversight/, showed that there have been significant failures in the organic meat, milk, eggs, and imported grains products on the part of the USDA. These markets are so large that buying from large-scale organic production farms again leaves the consumer open to the same fraud as without a third-party reviewer. Some products are marketed, presented, and sold as organic despite not following the regulations with inexpensive nonorganic agricultural inputs. The organic expectation by the consumer is that of a higher quality food product, but, unfortunately, these larger supply chains are sometimes challenging to track down and left open to the efficiencies and challenges of capitalism, making more money with less. Therefore, the integrity of the label

---

[39] Pollen, M. *Food Rules: An Eater's Guide,* December 2009.

has become somewhat doubtful. Again, one more reason to support your local, organic regenerative farmers.

Hidden Label Ingredients

Additives and preservatives are everywhere in processed foods. They help with shelf life, reduce food costs, provide a more visually pleasing product, and sweeten and change the texture of our foods. What they don't tell you is that they also contribute to disruptions in the microbiome. For those unfamiliar with the microbiome, it's essentially the bacteria, yeast, and fungi that live in our digestive tracts. The microbiome is important because it helps to maintain our health, and when it becomes out of kilter or a portion of it becomes unbalanced, so does our health. I'll go into this more in Chapter 7.

One of the most profound and immediate examples I've seen to date was published in *Nature Magazine,* entitled "Dietary Trehalose Enhances Virulence Of Epidemic *Clostridium Difficile*" by Collins et al., regarding a food additive called trehalose.[40] Trehalose is used commonly in ice cream as a substitute for sucrose or a form of sugar. Researchers found that small amounts of trehalose supported the growth of some of the more severe strains of Clostridium Difficile or C Diff that perhaps already existed within the GI tract of an individual but are, on the whole, outperformed by other members of the microbiome and doesn't generally cause problems. When C Diff has the opportunity to overgrow in the digestive tract because it's fed trehalose or there is some other imbalance, it can now overcome the competition. C diff is a particularly painful gastrointestinal disturbance that tends to manifest more in the immunocompromised and elderly as well as those taking antibiotics or antacids. It can cause inflammation from the toxins that it produces as well as a severe case of diarrhea that can last for weeks at a time. Anyone who has had C diff doesn't forget the experience nor do they want to experience it again.

---

[40] Collins, J. et al. Dietary Trehalose Enhances Virulence of Epidemic *Clostridium Difficile. Nature 553*, 291–294 (2018). https://doi.org/10.1038/nature25178

While this example may be considered extreme, the disruptions that food additives create on our microbiome aren't uncommon. Other examples include BispholA (BPA)and its analogs, Polychlorinated Biphenyls (PCB), parabens, heavy metals, triclosan, triclocarban, emulsifiers, and phthalates. And there are many more. While I could go into the direct impact on the microbiome of each of these, the important thing to understand is that any additive in a food product is put there for a purpose. Regardless of whether that purpose was well-intended, say to increase shelf life or make that product more appealing in some way, it doesn't mean it doesn't have a substantial negative health impact. The understanding needs to be that the removal of these from our diets as much as possible decreases the strain or total burden on our bodies to have to metabolize them. This increases the likelihood that our microbiomes will be less challenged to maintain a healthy balance. This, in cooperation with choosing foods that are regeneratively raised increases the likelihood that the microbiome will remain intact because the biome of the soil is doing some of that detoxing for you.

Local regenerative food producers provide healthier options. This is why I advocate for eating foods that don't have food labels added to them. Fresh food doesn't have the additives, preservatives, and artificial colors in them that we previously talked about. I also advocate for supporting local producers because many of them produce food because of a strong desire to ensure that healthy food options are available to them, their families, and the community. A local producer may seek to obtain one or more of the certifications previously listed in an effort to provide the consumer some assurance that what they're purchasing is, in fact, what is promoted. With any certifications, there are limitations to the process, so keep in mind that if a producer has more than one certification, this can provide a higher level of assuredness that you'll know what you're eating.

Talking With Your Local Producer

In the event that labels or certifications are completely not available, learn how to talk with your local food producers. Many farmers understand how a food is raised or grown has an impact on the health of the consumer, and they choose their methods based on this understanding. Some choose to forgo certifications due to the expense of certification. A producer that's proud of the way they're contributing to the food supply is happy to discuss practices that fostered their end product. Consider the following questions as examples:

What foods will you have in the coming weeks? This will help you prepare in advance for some great meals! With regard to sheep, cattle, bison, are your animals raised on pasture? Yes is best 100% of the time. Any grain fed the animals can change their fatty acid composition toward higher Omega 6. If so, for how long and when? Pasture raised or grass-fed animals retain a more health beneficial omega 3 (anti-inflammatory) to Omega 6 (pro-inflammatory) ratio. Are your animals ever fed grain that's not natural to its environment? If grain fed, even for a short time prior to processing, health benefits will be diminished. Sometimes, in winter months, producers may offer their animals hay, kelp, and other amendments. Ask if they're organic/regenerative as well. Do you use antibiotics in animal husbandry? Antibiotic residues can be found in meat products and have the likelihood of altering the consumers' gut microbial flora if eaten. Some producers will provide antibiotics just when animals are sick and then take that animal out of consideration for processing until it has been metabolized through their system. How do you control for insects and weeds? Are there circumstances in which you do use pesticides? Ideally, farmers will be using regenerative practices such as integrated pest management, cover crops, or biological testing and biological amending of the soil. Pesticide residues on produce are known endocrine disruptors, which have the potential of influencing endocrine, estrogen, thyroid, and neurotransmitters. Do you hold on-farm events? If so, how often and are they open to the public? Many producers will hold farm-to-table events or farm tours that showcase what they're about. Don't be afraid to go for a visit!

Local foods can be found not only at farmers' markets but also at other grocery stores that have an interest in supporting local or healthier food options. Keep an eye out for local food availability and even ask your local grocer if they carry any local/organic/grassfed/free-range/pasture-raised food products. If there's enough of a demand, the grocery store you frequent will eventually respond to your requests because they want your business. Local farmers' markets are also a great way to support local fresh food availability. COVID-19 disrupted our industrial supply chains to a tremendous degree. This would be one more reason to support local and build a relationship with the person who produces your food.

Other Sources for Help: Studies and Reviews

Other studies and reviews of food can also help to guide our decision making about what to put in our bodies. Studies that are worked in cooperation with a basic understanding of what goes into the production of our food can go a long way to guiding our food choices in a healthy way. The studies on oats products were a profound example of pesticide residues in oats that otherwise would have been a reasonably healthy food option. Another great example is the Oceana study on fish fraud in the American food supply.

As a dietitian, I'm consistently promoting high quality Omega 3 fatty acid sources, and fatty fish are a great source of highly bioavailable Omega 3s. So, when a study is done that basically indicates that more than 90% of fish is imported in this country, less than 1% is actually inspected for fraud, and that one third of the fish provided in grocery stores and restaurants is in fact mislabeled, it concerns me. They collected 1,200 samples from 674 retail outlets (grocery stores, restaurants and sushi venues) in 21 states. Seventy-four percent of fish in sushi venues are mislabeled.[41] This is another substantial failure at food transparency in our country.

In practice, I still encourage fish consumption from salmon, mackerel, sardines, and anchovies. These fish products tend to have fewer heavy metals in them despite some of them being pretty far down on the food chain. The bioaccumulation of heavy metals is a great concern and the reason why tuna didn't make this list. It tends to be quite high in mercury and heavily consumed. When

---

[41] Warner, K., Walker, T. Lowell, B., & Hirshfield, M. Oceana Study Reveals Seafood Fraud Nationwide, February 2013. https://oceana.org/wp-content/uploads/sites/18/National_Seafood_Fraud_Testing_Results_FINAL.pdf

the FDA has to provide warnings to the general public or to pregnant women about how much to eat of what, I tend to avoid the food product. Remember, in the ocean as well as on the land, we are what we eat but also what it eats. I also encourage people toward 100% grass-fed meats of any kind, including beef, lamb, and bison or wild game to get their Omega 3s. Walnuts, almonds, flax and chia seeds are also high in Omega 3 fatty acids but the bioavailability of the Omega 3s in meats is greater than in non-meat products so finding healthy meat-based options to avoid supplementation is important. It's not that supplements are bad per se, but choosing well comes with its own set of concerns that will be addressed further in Chapter 7

To take this a step further, it's not just fish that's not inspected when imported into America. The FDA has limited resources to inspect food imported into our country and, per the USDA ERS website, inspect approximately 1% of the 60 million tons of food under its regulatory authority for adulteration or misbranding.[42] To be clear, that's 59.4 million tons that aren't inspected. The inspections are anything but random and targeted at origins most likely to cause the greatest risk to human health. This means targeting routine offenders of import laws. All import refusals are reported under the FDA's Operational and Administrative System for Import Support (OASIS) database. The most common countries with food refusals are Mexico, India, and China. Most common foods refused are Fish/Seafood products, Vegetable/Vegetable Products, and Fruit/Fruit products. Approximately 19% of total food consumed in the United States is imported, including approximately 97% of fish and shellfish, approximately 50% of fresh fruits, and approximately 20% of fresh vegetables.[43] Not surprisingly, a study done on outbreaks of foodborne illness from 1996 to 2014 on imported foods indicate that the FDA's focus on a particular country and food products is

[42] USDA, ERS, Chart of imports refused. https://www.ers.usda.gov/webdocs/charts/62952/march16_feature_bovay_fig01.png?v=3607.7

[43] Bovay, J. FDA Refusals of Imported Food Products by Country and Category, 2005–2013, EIB-151, U.S. Department of Agriculture, Economic Research Service, March 2016. https://www.ers.usda.gov/webdocs/publications/44066/57014_eib151.pdf?v=0

warranted. During that time, 195 outbreaks of foodborne illness were studied which accounted for 10,685 illnesses, 1017 hospitalizations and 19 deaths with the most common foods contributing to these illnesses being seafood and produce.[44] [45] The most common pathogens involved were Salmonella and Cyclospora accounting for 75% of the illnesses with Mexico taking the lead on the origin of these illnesses. Where and in what capacity are outbreaks occurring? The FDA refused 87,552 shipments from 2005-2013 with 57,674 incidences of misbranding and 80,825 incidences of adulteration. They haven't exactly been relaxing on their laurels.

The question then becomes, what about the other 59.4 million tons? There are, no doubt, food products causing illness sliding under the radar because we don't know what we're eating. Remember the pasta example? An **adulterated** food per the Federal Food and Cosmetic Act of 1938 is one that contains, for example, poisonous ingredients, disease-causing bacteria, and viruses (pathogens), unsafe color additives, pesticide residues, or apparent filth. Per the same Act, a food is **misbranded** if it bears a false or misleading label with regard to ingredients, origin/manufacturer, or quality of ingredients. It's a little scary to think about food fraud happening on this scale.

Food fraud is rampant in America, and some of the most common foods that are adulterated in rank order include olive oil, milk, honey, saffron, coffee, maple syrup, orange juice, and grape wines.[46] As a dietitian, olive oil at the top of the list is very concerning. Frequently, I recommend eating more healthy fats.

---

[44] Gould, L. et al. Outbreaks of Disease Associated with Food Imported into the United States, 1996–2014. *Emerging Infectious Diseases.* 2017; *23*(3): 525-528. https://wwwnc.cdc.gov/eid/article/23/3/16-1462_article

[45] CDC, Table of Disease Outbreak. https://wwwnc.cdc.gov/eid/article/23/3/16-1462-t1

[46] Moore, J. C., Spink, J., & Lipp, M. Development and Application of a Database of Food Ingredient Fraud and Economically Motivated Adulteration from 1980 to 2010. *Journal of Food Science.* 2012 Apr; *77*(4) https://www.ncbi.nlm.nih.gov/pubmed/22486545

Remember that MD diet? Quite frankly it's hard to guide my clientele who some-times come from other parts of the country as well as other countries. Dare I say that the average American has never tried real, unadulterated, fresh olive oil and wouldn't know what to look for? The long and short of it comes down to a few simple things that help to skew the curve toward consumer confidence in buying. Always buy EVOO or extra virgin olive oil. Look for third-party certification such as the California Olive Oil Council (COOC), or the European Union's Protected Designation of Origin (PDO) which is the name of a geographical region or specific area that's recognized by official rules to produce certain foods with special characteristics related to location. If it's from Australia or Chile, buy it. They have much stricter regulations than other countries. These recommendations come from Tom Mueller's Book, *Extra Virginity*.[47] He also suggests that much of the olive oil is simply older oil that has been mixed with newer oil and then sold as fresh olive oil. From a health standpoint, we don't need to eat old oil that has had an opportunity to go rancid as this is an oxidative process as well as a process that reduces some of the nutritive properties of the oil itself. Not to mention it simply just makes it taste bad.

Another example that didn't make the top 10 list but is near and dear to my heart is parmesan cheese. True Italian Parmigiano Reggiano made from grass-fed cow milk is so delicious that once you have had it you'll never go back. If you want to purchase the real thing, look for cheese that has been cut into sections at the cheese department that still has the casing on it. You'll be able to see portions of the wording, Parmigiano Reggiano, which is a PDO but the word Parmesan is used across the board in America. Do not buy pre shredded if you want the real thing. It's a hard cheese that crumbles in your hand when pressed and has tyrosine flavor crystals that literally melt in your mouth when you eat it. Most parmesan cheese isn't real Parmesan and, in this country, we like to add wood pulp to make a little cheese go a longer way. Not a palatable easy to digest filler option to say the least.

---

[47] Mueller, T. *Extra Virginity*, 2011.

Adulteration of food or miss marketing isn't a new thing in America. It has been going on for decades. Here is a link to America's Chamber of Horrors: https://www.fda.gov/about-fda/virtual-exhibits-fda-history/80-years-federal-food-drug-and-cosmetic-act. It shows some of the interesting, almost entertaining approaches that food and supplement manufacturers have taken over the years for historical perspective on the promotion of food products. This subject could be a whole other book!

Do Your Best With the Information You Have

Many more examples could be provided here within these pages, but the message ultimately needs to be one of encouragement. One that empowers the average consumer to make wiser food choices in an effort to support health. If we generally choose foods that don't have a label, have been sourced locally from a farmer who has an interest in using sustainable, regenerative, or organic agricultural practices, and we cook at home, we're making strides in a healthier direction. Arguably, cooking at home more often could be the single most important action to encourage health. This allows us to ensure we're taking charge of our food environments, taking charge of what we're putting in our bodies, and perhaps leading our healthiest life possible.

While this chapter may have seemed a bit overwhelming with information about how little we really know about our food, in clinical practice, I tell people to do the best they can with what they do know. Educate or arm yourself with as much information as you reasonably can digest and choose foods wisely. There's no way for everyone to know everything about what we have available to us in the grocery store or other markets. Write down a few simple things you could do the next time before you head to the grocery store and implement changes over a week or few weeks. Maybe it's reading food labels more frequently, buying more fruits and vegetables, or just choosing more organic foods. Maybe it's going to the farmers' market for the first time, starting a garden, trying a new recipe, or visiting with Suzie and Fred down the road who have a farm stand you drive by every day but have never stopped at. Any of these options take an all-important step toward connecting you more closely with your food and making wiser choices.

5.
The Tornado that Tore Through our World Wide Food System

What happens when we can't eat at home because our food supply has been cut off due to a major worldwide catastrophe or because we're too afraid to go to the grocery store? This is what the COVID-19 crisis functionally did to us and our food system. It illustrates the dysfunctionality of the system quite nicely. On March 13, 2020, our president declared a national public health emergency. Regardless of political affiliation, whether you subscribe to the conspiracy theory behind COVID-19 or believe that it was a naturally occurring event, are Republican, Democrat, or Independent, the result is the same. Ten out of ten people need to eat. Our food system during this crisis became additionally broken.

To be clear, the brokenness of our food system wasn't because there was no food available. There have been hundreds of accounts of produce being tilled back into the ground, milk poured out onto fields or animal meat products brought to slaughter and composted. It's because the routine supply chains that deliver the food were additionally broken and there was very little effort to find alternative routes or outlets as well as the fact that processing facilities for food were also impaired due to worker sickness. For some reason, processing facilities seemed to be a hot bed for breeding COVID infections; whether it was because of conditions within the facilities or community contact still remains to be completely determined.

As of July 10, 2020, 16,233 cases of COVID had been reported in 239 processing facilities across 23 states.[48] 87% of cases infected racial or ethnic minorities. It has been theorized that some of the infections didn't occur within the facility itself but in the close quarters of some of the homes of workers with large families and in close quarters with transportation to and from the facilities. This coupled with the work environment within a processing facility, close contact within the processing plant for longer than 15 minutes at a time and other shared workspaces allowed for the spread. Additionally, if one thinks about what a processing facility is, it doesn't take too much of an imagination to envision DNA flying through the air waiting for a virus to attach itself to it. Despite the federal mandate to remain open, these facilities became hot beds for the virus and were forced to close.

Some of the facilities were closed by management and others closed by the local health departments as a matter of public safety. The result, as most of these facilities are in rural counties, was the short-term layoff of thousands of people who sometimes live paycheck to paycheck. The additional consequence of these closures was that the larger meat producers were now looking for ways to process products with their own facilities closed. The result was that the larger meat producers ended up scheduling with the smaller local processors in an attempt to keep up with demand for their products.

Now in local food circles, we consistently hear about the small producer who makes it into the larger markets only to be undercut by a larger producer for a short time with a sale and then put out of business. While the larger producer's product is flying off the shelf, the smaller producer's product sits on the shelf because it costs four to five times more during that sale period. The relationships the smaller producers have with their customer base keeps customers coming back year after year. What's happening this time is quite different. Prior to COVID–19, it didn't make financial sense for these large meat producers to

---

[48] CDC Morbidity and Mortality Weekly. Update: COVID-19 Among Workers in Meat and Poultry Processing Facilities — United States, April–May 2020, July 10, 2020 / 69(27): 887-892 https://www.cdc.gov/mmwr/volumes/69/wr/mm6927e2.htm

attempt processing at a small facility. But during COVID, they had no choice. In talking with three of our more successful small meat producers, I heard the same story over and over. There was plenty of demand for their product but no way to have it processed. The result is the same. The small producer goes out of business because there are no processing dates until 2022, as the dates had been booked by larger producers for several years. It was a quick, sad end for some.

Big Ag Has Not Suffered During COVID

Most meat production and processing in America is owned by foreign countries. JBS of Brazil is the largest processor in the world of pork and beef. Smithfield, owned by WH group of China, owns many facilities and their Sioux Falls facility accounts for 4-5% of our country's pork production. Tyson says right on their website that they produce 20% of the beef, pork, and chicken in our country but if one looks into who owns Tyson, it becomes very quickly quite complicated to the average consumer. Tyson has approximately 57 legal operating entities and subsidiaries. Most are American but many are not, so, while technically initially an American company, much of the sales, processing and distribution is accomplished by non-American companies. How could they have responded to a COVID 19 pandemic? Unless they had local supply chains set up, they couldn't have responded. Foreign-owned companies that don't have a vested interest in local communities wouldn't even know where to start.

This coupled with the fact that JBS set sales records in 2021[49], with overall net sales increasing by 20.7% in the midst of a pandemic and rising meat prices, should raise some eyebrows. The company claims that the reason is because the Swine Flu, which reduced the pig population by 40% in China, preceded COVID concerns. Exports to China almost doubled in revenue, recording

---

[49] Sims, B., & Shaffer, E. JBS Sets Record Earning, *Meat and Poultry*, 03.27.2020 https://www.meatpoultry.com/articles/22838-jbs-sets-earnings-record-in-2019#:~:-text=JBS%20Brazil%2C%20which%20includes%20leather,in%20the%20quarter%2C%20JBS%20said.

increases of 61% in volume and 23% in prices. Meanwhile, our shelves are bare or we're paying $25.00 for a 4 pack of pork chops with price gouging running rampant.

Tyson sales grew only 6% in 2019. Overall numbers were impacted by a variety of business expenses but, most interestingly, by the acquisition of Keystone Foods in 2018 and Thai and European Operations. Keystone Foods has eight plants and three innovation centers in China, South Korea, Malaysia, Thailand, and Australia as well as six processing plants in Alabama, Georgia, Kentucky, North Carolina, Pennsylvania, and Wisconsin. The Thai and European Operations purchased in 2019 includes four processing facilities in Thailand, one processing facility in the Netherlands, and one processing facility in the United Kingdom. This is a gigantic conglomerate. This isn't local food even if you have one of these plants in your backyard. These are the plants that may help a local economy by bringing jobs to a particular location, but, ultimately, very little of the money actually stays where these facilities are located.

I don't advocate for their products in any way. These examples are for folks to understand that the industrialized food system needs to be dismantled or, at least, not supported by the American consumer when it comes to products that can be produced locally. They produce large volumes of less healthy food products that negatively impact communities and our environment. These are the companies that support CAFO development, run large semis up and down rural roads, diminish air quality, and pollute the local water.

Bringing It Back Home

Meanwhile, in SW Missouri during COVID-19, people were frequenting farmer markets and local producers were concerned they could meet enough of the demand because of their own record sales. And no, they didn't charge more for their products. They could have but chose not to because their relationship with the customer was too important to them. They couldn't have predicted the COVID-19 virus and, even if they had a crystal ball, couldn't respond to the needs of the local food system that quickly. By late October 2019, we Americans had some idea of the potential magnitude of the COVID-19 problem and by early March 2020 the country was shut down. Basically, it was four months from start to shut down and we in 2023 are still muddling through the fallout.

We Americans were quite spoiled when it comes to food availability prior to the shutdown. We go to the grocery store and pick up what we want to have for dinner that evening. Meanwhile, the local meat producer is planning 9 months to 2 years in advance to ensure availability of meat products. Plant or fruit and vegetable producers are planning at least several months to a year in advance. Conversely, had we been purchasing local food products year-round and consistently, it would have ensured larger volumes of food product availability with no likelihood that any of it would be shipped to China. This is why the food was still available at the farmers' markets.

Historically speaking, the loss of the diversified farm in favor of a single bottom line that's strictly about efficiency and economies of scale driving animal and food production *IS* the problem. When three foreign-owned companies own 80% of the meat market in America, we have a serious problem on our hands. When 10 companies own 75% of the shelved food market (more on this in the next chapter), we have yet another problem. These models of efficiency have destroyed small business (community), food safety, food security, jobs, access to information about our food and food system, and small farmer independence. There has to be consideration for our rural communities and small farmers as well as the environment but there's very little policy that supports all three.

There are organizations attempting to pull all three together. Organizations like R-CALF USA this year were successful in gaining over 250,000 signatures on MCOOL or Mandatory Country of Origin Labeling petitioning our government. Their petition supports all three: the small farmer, rural communities, and the environment: https://www.r-calfusa.com/ranch-groups-mandatory-country-of-origin-labeling-petition-gains-250k-signatures-in-7-days/. MCOOL will aid in national food security and stimulate the USA's economic growth. How would MCOOL do this? Food Transparency. Americans should be allowed to know where the meat that they're eating is born, raised, and processed. As illustrated above, it would be almost impossible to know given that most of our food is no longer from American companies. Unfortunately, MCOOL remains repealed.

Relaxing of Labeling Standards During COVID Potentially Sacrifices Health

In the midst of the pandemic, the FDA decided to relax labeling of food products and menu labeling standards to accommodate some of the concerns with food supply chains. On the surface, that appears to be quite altruistic and supportive of the industrialized food industry, but fundamentally, what it actually does is undermine food safety at its core. As indicated previously, these companies weren't suffering during COVID.

I couldn't say it better than the FDA:

> "Given this public health emergency, and as discussed in the Notice in the Federal Register of March 25, 2020, titled "Process for Making Available Guidance Documents Related to Coronavirus Disease 2019," available at https://www.govinfo.gov/content/pkg/FR-2020-03- 25/pdf/2020-06222.pdf, this guidance is being implemented without prior public comment because FDA has determined that prior public participation for this guidance is not feasible or appropriate (see section 701(h)(1)(C) of the FD&C Act (21 U.S.C. 371(h)(1)(C)) and 21 CFR 10.115(g)(2)). This guidance document is being implemented immediately, but it remains subject to comment in accordance with our good guidance practices."[50]

---

[50] Temporary Policy Regarding Certain Food Labeling Requirements During the COVID-19 Public Health Emergency: Minor Formulation Changes and Vending Machines Guidance for Industry May 2020 U.S. Department of Health and Human Services Food and Drug Administration Center for Food Safety and Applied Nutrition/Office of Nutrition and Food Labeling. https://www.fda.gov/media/138315/download

Their responsiveness was quite impressive given that the pandemic wasn't actually recognized until March 13, 2020. As they stated, the decision was made *without* public comment as the FDA didn't find it feasible or appropriate. To dive a little further into this issue to understand its significance, again, I couldn't say it better than the FDA:

> "FDA is issuing this guidance to food manufacturers to provide temporary and limited flexibilities in food labeling requirements under certain circumstances. Our goal is to provide regulatory flexibility, where fitting, to help minimize the impact of supply chain disruptions associated with the current COVID-19 pandemic on product availability. For example, we are providing flexibility for manufacturers to use existing labels, without making otherwise required changes, when making minor formula adjustments due to unforeseen shortages or supply chain disruptions brought about by the COVID-19 pandemic."[50]

This means that manufacturers don't have to disclose what they're feeding you and won't get in trouble for it. If one reads the fine print of the document that the FDA provided, there cannot be any substitutions of the major food allergens including fish, shellfish, dairy, soy, wheat, peanuts, tree nuts, and eggs, which account for 90% of all food allergies. Food manufacturers are allowed to substitute pretty much anything else and without recourse from the consumer should someone become ill. As a professional who works quite closely with people who have food allergies, this is inexcusable for the following reasons:

1. Supply chains that have been broken are generally not the ones whose food ingredients would be substituted.

2. 160 foods have been identified as food allergens. This leaves 152 ingredients that can be mislabeled according to the FDA.

3. The other 10% of recognized allergens aren't listed in the document and only covered as "probable" allergens. If 32 million people have identified allergies, this leaves 3.2 million people without

recourse if they eat something to which they're allergic because of an unidentified allergen.

4. Every year, 175,000 people require emergency room visits to manage food allergic reactions already. This does not include those who manage it at home and with more restrictive food labeling.

With some labeling requirements being lifted, the potential for anaphylactic reactions or reactions that require hospitalization are much more likely to occur. To what degree this could happen remains unknown. If one were to weigh the relative risk of dying from COVID-19 versus mislabeling a food product, I personally would take my chances with COVID-19 because I can take more charge over my exposure and support my immune system by eating well. This is one of the many reasons I encourage my clients towards food that has no label and is grown or raised regeneratively. We don't know what we're eating and the most recent action from the FDA has provided us even less food transparency. This action was supposed to remain in effect until November of 2023. What guarantee does the consumer have that the industry will revert back to previous food labeling laws?

How Do We Circumnavigate Big Ag? Food Sovereignty

With all of this being said about what has become known about the multinational corporations or Big Ag that are in charge of approximately 90% of our food supply, the next question then becomes, how do we take back charge of our food supply? And does it make sense to do so?

In local food circles, there's much discussion around the concept of food sovereignty. Food sovereignty is the food system in which people who produce the food are also in charge of the policies of food production as well as its distribution. This is pretty much how it is on the island of Vitality and the very reason why producing food on some level is so important. The more self-reliant we consumers or "eaters" become, the less important it is that at-home food prices went up 6.3% in 2021 and in 2022 were up 10.4%, according to the USDA

Economic Research Service. If we're food sovereign, we aren't eating many of these industrialized foods to begin with. There may be some changes in agricultural inputs, such as the cost of diesel, that impact overall pricing in an area that has achieved food sovereignty but, for the most part, let the prices rise in the regular markets. Local food security has the capability of translating to supporting a local food economy that's not entirely but quite separate from many of these other influences.

As previously discussed, the current system is artificially propped up to put money in the pockets of these multinational corporations. If funding or the Farm Bill were removed, there's no telling what might happen to the current food system. While the claims are false that we're feeding the world, we're producing a lot of foods or at least food-like substances that most people still eat. Are there enough sustainable or regenerative agricultural products to feed us? No. Not likely and distribution chains aren't fully set up either. This doesn't negate the responsibility to begin to move in that direction, and as consumers start thinking in the context of how we spend our money and therefore dictate what continues to be available on the market. For those more inclined to grow food, start thinking in terms of local food systems and plan ahead for the next supply chain issue that may collapse. This is heady stuff but not so far out there. We have experienced it for the past three years already.

Many organizations both national and international now focus on support for the family farm and local food systems in combination with encouragement toward regenerative agriculture or, at least, organic agriculture. Here is a link to a list of 119 organizations shaking up the food system in 2019: https://foodtank.com/news/2019/01/119-organizations-to-watch-in-2019/. Keep in mind that, on some level, during COVID, the small producer helped to feed our communities. It's not so far out there to imagine that this could be done on a larger scale for a longer term if approached intentionally.

6.
Which Roadmap to Vitality Do I Choose?

Have you ever decided to go on a road trip so you go into your glove box, pull out this old map that back in the day was super useful to get you from point A to point B? But now you realize with technological advances and Google maps that pretty much no one reads a map anymore. We all have smart phones so we rely on technology spouting directions from the Bluetooth on the console rather than the old-fashioned way of becoming in touch with north, south, east, and west with a topographical or other physical map. On some occasions, Google maps will actually send you around in circles. This is the same problem that we have with nutrition information overload. We have so much information at our fingertips, yet we've lost our direction.

There's an overwhelming amount of nutrition information out there on the market, and I'm not going to attempt to unravel it in this chapter or even recommend which diet book to follow. Certain understandings about basic general good health relating to nutrition need to be identified and followed in order to influence overall health, no matter what ails you. A key concept to keep in mind is that we aren't victims of our genetics. Over the years, I've had a multitude of my clients tell me that they just have bad genes and they throw their hands up in despair and decide that any effort that they make toward improving their health situation will be fruitless. After all, Mom or Dad were overweight. Why should there be any other expectation? On the contrary, we are closer to 10% our genes and 90% our environments, which include diet, lifestyle, socialization, exercise, the air we breathe, and the products we put on our skin. So, making positive modifications to any of these will help to improve health incrementally.

There is, in fact, a multigenerational influence at play, which should motivate at least the child-bearing generation. Functionally, that is to say, how we treat our own bodies has an influence on even our grandchildren. So, while you may not have been set up for success by your parents or grandparents, it doesn't mean that the changes you make are without merit, even though you may not be seeing the direct, immediate impacts you strive for. There is a generational or epigenetic "hangover" of chosen lifestyles that are then attributed to bad genes rather than bad choices or food environments. These generally take several generations to correct but when looking at it from the 20,000-foot view, any positive change is inching the needle in the right direction. In America, we're overfed with calories but undernourished because of large-scale availability of food that's not supporting our health. All is very far from lost, however.

Agricultural Practices Really Do Matter

To discuss the basic premise about nutrition recommendations, I must first discuss agricultural practices and why they matter. Remember, food is agriculture. Agricultural practices are important when it comes to not only personal health but the health of our communities and environments. The quality of the end product is distinctly different relative to whether a food was grown or raised organically, regeneratively, or conventionally. Conventionally raised foods are the makings of our industrialized food system. They're the foods that are mostly available to us, feed into the system of convenience, tend to be highly processed, have lower nutrient values, and foster our ill health. They are the things one should eat the least.

A review article by Davis, entitled "Declining Fruit and Vegetable Nutrient Composition: What Is the Evidence?"[51] indicates that the micronutrient and mineral values of different food products may have, in fact, diminished over time and that higher yields may sacrifice nutritional quality. Another publication entitled *Changes in USDA Food Composition Data for 43 Garden Crops, 1950 to 1999*, really upset the proverbial apple cart when it suggested that there had been a major decline in nutrient values for 43 crops.[52] While nutrient values have certainly dropped on some level because of our farming practices, we must be cautious with the interpretation also because the science behind determining nutrient values has changed in the 49 years between studies. The way the testing is accomplished is different. This means that we may be comparing apples to oranges on some level. The initial publication even indicates that some of the differences could be due to the difference in varieties of what was tested as well. We produce fewer varieties or diversity of every food now versus 50 years ago. This is, in part, because our industrialized food system favors crops with more weather tolerant traits and higher yield monocrops.

However, Antione Lavoisier taught us in 1785 that through the Law of Conservation of Mass, matter cannot be created or destroyed. It can only change form or, in the case of agriculture, form and sometimes location, specifically downstream. For example, there's a finite amount of calcium, iron, phosphorus, and other minerals on the planet. So, if our agricultural inputs to conventionally raised crops only add back what's known as NPK (Nitrogen, Phosphorus, Potassium) fertilizers with very few other amendments it stands to reason that it will become depleted eventually of the amendments that aren't added back. Our soil contains so much more than just nitrogen, phosphorus,

---

[51] Davis, D. R. (2009). Declining Fruit and Vegetable Nutrient Composition: What Is the Evidence?, *HortScience 44*(1), 15-19. http://saveoursoils.com/userfiles/downloads/1351255687-Changes%20in%20USDA%20food%20composition%20data%20for%2043%20garden%20crops,%201950-1999.pdf

[52] Davis, D. R., Epp, M. D., & Riordan, H.D. Changes in USDA Food Composition Data for 43 Garden Crops, 1950 to 1999. *Journal of the American College of Nutrition*. 2004 Dec; *23*(6): 669-82. https://pubmed.ncbi.nlm.nih.gov/15637215/

and potassium, so, with these being the major three nutrients added back to the soil, it might ultimately fail to grow food at some point because a plant cannot just continue to take from the soil or is it just produces lower quality end products like the study suggested. This is not an accurate representation of the problem, however. The problem is more that these amendments impact the microbiome of the soil, which in turn impacts the nutrients and nutrient availability of what is in the soil.

The soil microbiome has its own complex little ecosystem down under the surface that supports a synergistic relationship between the bacteria, fungi, yeast, minerals, other micronutrients, and the plants that reside there much like the microbiomes in our own gastrointestinal tracts. Without healthy soil, our plants and animals cannot be as healthy as they would be otherwise because the nutrient quality of the soil has diminished, as the larger biome is no longer present. Without a healthy biome of the soil, the plants don't have a plant-available form of nutrition in the soil to access. So, on some level, the previous studies are accurate in the sense that the plants don't contain the same nutrition because they cannot access it. Where the land has been treated with conventional agricultural practices, organic matter and biology would have to be purposefully replaced in order for the plants to be full of the nutrients and minerals again that they were previously able to pull from the soil.

Many studies have been done on the nutrient compositions and, in particular, phytochemical concentration, of organic vs. regenerative vs. conventional agriculture. For example, a study done by Tarrozi et al. in 2006 "clearly show that organic red oranges have a higher phytochemical content (i.e., phenolics, anthocyanins and ascorbic acid), total antioxidant activity and bioactivity than integrated red oranges."[53] A review article by Worthington, entitled "Effect of Agricultural Methods on Nutritional Quality: A Comparison of Organic With Conventional

---

[53] Tarozzi, A., Hrelia, S., Angeloni, C., Morroni, F., Biagi, P., Guardigli, M., Cantelli-Forti, G., & Hrelia, P. Antioxidant Effectiveness of Organically and Non-Organically Grown Red Oranges in Cell Culture Systems. *European Journal of Nutrition*. 2006 Mar; 45(3):152-158. https://www.ncbi.nlm.nih.gov/pubmed/16096701

Crops" reviewed literature over the last 50 years.[54] On the whole, the review shows higher nutrient values and lower nitrate values for organic crops. Depending on the crop, studies have shown statistically significant higher flavonoid, polyphenol, anthocyanin, ascorbic acid, citric acid, and alpha tocopherol concentrations for those raised regeneratively or organically. Another study by Stazi in 2018 showed an increased ability of plants to take up iron as well as diminished uptake of arsenic from the soil in tomatoes under organic conditions,[55] or in essence, leaving heavy metals behind.[56] Iron is desirable to have in the food supply while arsenic is not. Heavy metals can be quite toxic to human beings. I'm not going to review all the articles referenced in the footnotes of this book, but it's important to note that this applies to many fruits and vegetables as well as tree crops. The articles referenced are to rice, eggplant, apples, potatoes, peaches, oranges, and pears when

---

[54] Worthington, V. Effect of Agricultural Methods on Nutritional Quality: A Comparison of Organic With Conventional Crops. *Alternative Therapies & Health Medicine*. 1998 Jan; *4*(1): 58-69. https://pubmed.ncbi.nlm.nih.gov/9439021/

[55] Stazi, S. R., Mancinelli, R., Marabottini, R., Allevato, E., Radicetti, E., Campiglia, E., & Marinari, S. Influence of Organic Management on As Bioavailability: Soil Quality and Tomato As Uptake. *Chemosphere*. 2018 Nov; *211*: 352-359. https://www.ncbi.nlm.nih.gov/pubmed/30077931

[56] Kumar Rai, P., Soo Lee, S., Zhang, M., Tsang, Y. F., & Kim, K-H. Heavy Metals in Food Crops: Health Risks, Fate, Mechanisms, and Management, *Environment International*, Volume 125, 2019, Pages 365-385, https://www.sciencedirect.com/science/article/pii/S0160412018327971?via%3Dihub

I stopped researching.[57] [58] [59] [60] [61] [62] [63] [64] It's not really a question that ultimately the end product is better for us; the question is in what way and to what degree?

[57] Akyol, H., Riciputi, Y., Capanoglu, E., Caboni, M. F., Verardo, V. Phenolic Compounds in the Potato and Its Byproducts: An Overview. *International Journal of Molecular Science.* 2016 May 27; *17*(6): 835. https://pubmed.ncbi.nlm.nih.gov/27240356/

[58] Carbonaro, M., Mattera, M., Nicoli, S., Bergamo, P., & Cappelloni, M. Modulation of Antioxidant Compounds in Organic vs. Conventional Fruit (Peach, Prunus Persica L., and Pear, Pyrus Communis L.). *Journal of Agricultural Food Chemistry.* 2002 Sep 11; *50*(19):5458-5462. https://www.ncbi.nlm.nih.gov/pubmed/12207491

[59] Fernandes, V. C., Domingues, V. F., de Freitas, V., Delerue-Matos, C., & Mateus, N. Strawberries from Integrated Pest Management and Organic Farming: Phenolic Composition and Antioxidant Properties. *Food Chemistry.* 2012 Oct 15; *134*(4):1926-1931. https://www.ncbi.nlm.nih.gov/pubmed/23442640

[60] Kaur, A. et al. Organic Cultivation of Ashwagandha with Improved Biomass and High Content of Active Withanolides: Use of Vermicompost. *PLoS One.* 2018 Apr 16; *13*(4): e0194314. https://www.ncbi.nlm.nih.gov/pubmed/29659590

[61] Kesarwani, A., Chiang, P. Y., Chen, S. S. Distribution of Phenolic Compounds and Antioxidative Activities of Rice Kernel and Their Relationships With Agronomic Practice. *Scientific World Journal. 2014*:620171. https://www.ncbi.nlm.nih.gov/pubmed/25506072

[62] Lombardi-Boccia, G., Lucarini, M., Lanzi, S., Aguzzi, A., Cappelloni, M. Nutrients and Antioxidant Molecules in Yellow Plums (Prunus Domestica L.) from Conventional and Organic Productions: A Comparative Study. *Journal Agricultural Food Chemistry.* 2004 Jan 14; *52*(1): 90-94. https://pubmed.ncbi.nlm.nih.gov/14709018/

[63] Virginia Worthington. Nutritional Quality of Organic Versus Conventional Fruits, Vegetables, and Grains. *The Journal of Alternative and Complementary Medicine.* Apr 2001.161-173. https://www.liebertpub.com/doi/abs/10.1089/107555301750164244

[64] Raigón, M. D., Rodríguez-Burruezo, A., & Prohens, J. Effects of Organic and Conventional Cultivation Methods on Composition of Eggplant Fruits. *Journal of*

Regenerative agriculture supports the plant cell structure, which creates an increase in phytochemicals and helps the plant fight off pests and disease as well. These foods have higher phytochemical content in part because the phytochemicals are associated with the plants' defense system. When no pesticides are applied, the plant can then support its own defense system via the good bacteria and fungi of the environment, much like our own body's immune system needs to be challenged in order to fend for itself and build its own immunity. When a plant doesn't have to do this, the phytochemical content drops and, in some cases, the protein content also drops. Here is the kicker, though. The soil biology has to be present during critical periods of growth for the plant to be able to do this. If the soil biology isn't there, the plant will again be open to attack and crops will still fail.

Phytochemicals can be found in all foods of plant origin. Different phytochemicals are usually identified in association with the different colors of the plants. Anthocyanins, like in cabbage, tend to be purple; certain types of polyphenols tend to vary between light green, yellow and red or black like in tea or cocoa powder; curcumin in turmeric tends to be bright orange; and so on. There are literally hundreds of these compounds associated with food. The important thing to remember is that these compounds tend to have high antioxidant capacity and help our bodies manage inflammation which helps to fight cancer as well as cardiovascular disease. So, eating our colors from the garden should be in order. It's also interesting to note that, sometimes, this can mean a better tasting end product. Have you ever tried an organic carrot vs a conventionally grown one? They're so much sweeter and more delicious. It's hard to improve on what mother nature provides in original packaging. When our land is managed regeneratively, we should perhaps leave mother nature to do her thing.

Agricultural Food Chemistry. 2010 Jun 9; *58*(11):6833-6840. https://www.ncbi.nlm.nih.gov/pubmed/20443597

Poopooing the Pesticide Panacea

Pesticides are defined as chemical substances that are used to prevent, destroy or mitigate any pests that may interfere with the growing of crop, including insects (insecticide), rodents (rodenticide), weeds (herbicide) or micro-organisms (algicide, fungicide or bactericide). The large-scale use of pesticides started in the 1930s and their use became quite widespread by the 1950s and was initially promoted along with fertilization as supporting greater yield for the farmers as part of the "Green Revolution." At the time, the promotion to the farmers was a case for less time, labor, fuel, and machinery needed for mechanical weed control. I saw an old promotion for the use of glyphosate indicating that using it would actually decrease the need for overall pesticide use.

The USDA Economic Research Service (ERS), in their 2014 report entitled *Pesticide Use in US Crops: 21 Selected Crops 1960-2008)* [65] tells the story of the dramatic rise in pesticide use in America. The 21 crops in the study included apples, barley, corn, cotton, grapefruit, grapes, lemons, lettuce, peaches, peanuts, pears, pecans, potatoes, oranges, rice, sorghum, soybeans, sugarcane, sweet corn, tomatoes, and wheat. These crops account for 72% of overall use of pesticides in America. The report covers the ins and outs of what kind was used where, but the point that I would like to emphasize here is this:

> "Rapid growth characterized the first 20 years, ending in 1981. The total quantity of pesticides applied to the 21 crops analyzed grew from 196 million pounds of pesticide active ingredients in 1960 to 632 million pounds in 1981. Improvements in the types and modes of action of active ingredients applied along with small annual fluctuations resulted in a slight downward trend in pesticide use to 516 million pounds in 2008."

[65] USDA Pesticide Use US Agriculture of 21 Selected Crops 1960-2008, *Economic Research Service Economic Information Bulletin* Number 124 ,May 2014. https://www.ers.usda.gov/webdocs/publications/43854/46734_eib124.pdf

So, for perspective, we went from zero pesticides to 196 million pounds in 1960? Landing at 516 million pounds in 2008 for just 21 crops? This is with current estimates of pesticide use at over a billion pounds used in the USA currently and 5.6 billion pounds used worldwide. Wait a minute. Wasn't the whole GMO market promoted as necessary to decrease pesticide usage?

There have been many studies showing that insecticides, pesticides, and herbicides are significantly more toxic with their adjuvants.[66] [67] [68]Adjuvants are the part of the formulations within the pesticides that are considered "inert" and, therefore, don't require testing for safety. One such ingredient in these formulations was considered inert as a pesticide but active as a cleaning agent. This makes no sense. We're concerned about cleaning with it, but is it fine to eat it? From a health standpoint, this is concerning because there's a disconnect between science and regulatory policy. Much of the promotion around glyphosate and other products are done just on the active ingredient, therefore, proving its safety in the eyes of the Environmental Protection Agency (EPA), the regulatory agency responsible for protecting human health associated with these chemicals. It's, therefore, important to note that in 100% of the cases, the formulations with "inert" ingredients amplify toxicity on human cells from 125-1,000 times![68]

Roundup, largely promoted due to its safety factors, is, in fact, "just" 125 times more toxic than glyphosate, its active ingredient. It's also the most widely used herbicide on the market and the chemical that Roundup-ready food science

[66] Mesnage, R., Defarge, N., Spiroux de Vendômois, J., & Séralini, G. E. Major Pesticides Are More Toxic to Human Cells Than Their Declared Active Principles. *Biomedical Research International*. 2014: 179691. https://pubmed.ncbi.nlm.nih.gov/24719846/?dopt=Abstract

[67] Mesnage, R., & Antoniou, M. N. Ignoring Adjuvant Toxicity Falsifies the Safety Profile of Commercial Pesticides. *Frontlines of Public Health*. 2018 Jan 22; *5*: 361. https://pubmed.ncbi.nlm.nih.gov/29404314/

[68] Janssens, L., Stoks, R., Stronger Effects of Roundup Than Its Active Ingredient Glyphosate in Damselfly Larvae. *Aquatic Toxicology*. 2017 Dec; *193*: 210-216. https://pubmed.ncbi.nlm.nih.gov/29100103/

has been developed around. Some of the top foods we subsidize in this country are also genetically modified such as 92% of corn and 94% of soy. Other crops that are Roundup-ready include canola, cotton (cottonseed oil), sugar beets, potato, squash, and papaya.

Roundup-ready crops only account for 56% of glyphosate usage[69], however. It's also used as a desiccant in certain parts of the country, which means it's sprayed on crops to dry them out even if they're not GMO. It's estimated that up to 70 different crops are influenced by this practice including corn, cotton, canola, soybeans, sugar beets, alfalfa, berry crops, brassica vegetables, bulb vegetables, fruiting vegetables, leafy vegetables, legume vegetables, cucurbit vegetables, root tuber vegetables, cereal grains, grain sorghum, citrus crops, fallow, herbs and spices, orchards, tropical and subtropical fruits, stone fruits, pome fruits, nuts, vine crops, oilseed crops, and sugarcane. This information comes straight from the FDA website.

The National Wheat Foundation indicates on their website that in 2016 "only" 33% of wheat in the US had glyphosate spread on their crops.[70] This is a high percentage for a crop that's also not genetically modified. Current EPA thresholds are set at a Maximum Contaminant Level (MCL) of 700 ppb and if levels were found above the tolerance level the commodity or food would be subject to seizure by the government. One might wonder what the overall exposure would be to glyphosate daily if considering total dietary intakes including cereal or grains like wheat and oats. Remember that our eating patterns in the United States are geared more towards these highly processed foods. And the Food Guide Pyramid promoted 6-11 servings of grains for almost 2 decades from

[69] Benbrook, C. M. Trends in Glyphosate Herbicide Use in the United States and Globally. *Environmental Science Europe.* 2016; *28*(1): 3. https://www.ncbi.nlm.nih.gov/pmc/articles/PMC5044953/

[70] National Wheat Foundation website. The Facts About Glyphosate, Part 1: How Do Wheat Growers Use Glyphosate?. https://wheatfoundation.org/the-truth-about-glyphosate-part-1-how-do-wheat-growers-use-glyphosate/

1992 to 2011. How much are our children eating relative to their body weights and how is this impacting their endocrine systems if not eating organically?

The Government Accountability Office (GAO) is an independent, nonpartisan agency that works for Congress. From their website, they're often called the "congressional watchdog." GAO examines how taxpayer dollars are spent and provides Congress and federal agencies with objective, reliable information to help the government save money and work more efficiently." In their 2014 publication entitled *FOOD SAFETY: FDA and USDA Should Strengthen Pesticide Residue Monitoring Programs and Further Disclose Monitoring Limitations*[71],they indicate that when food is tested, many times it's not tested for commonly used pesticides, including glyphosate, with established tolerance levels. This isn't disclosed in their reporting. How is this possible? The most commonly used pesticide isn't even tested for? Why set a limit if it's not even going to be tracked? Finally, in 2016, the FDA started testing for glyphosate, a good 45 years after it was placed on the market.

Also, the FDA doesn't use statistically valid methods consistent with the Office of Management and Budget (OMB) standards to collect national information on the incidence and level of pesticide residues. This makes the data that's available next to impossible to interpret. I went in search of such data which is easily found in a text-like spreadsheet format with hundreds of potential contaminants listed in different food products such as milk, low fat milk, chocolate milk, cheese, ground beef, ham, pork, etc. Literally hundreds of tests of the same food products, one has to scroll down through in order to find the product of concern. The only way to find the information is to scroll through thousands upon thousands of entries and keep scrolling. Did I mention how much you have to scroll? It was cumbersome to say the least. In this day of technology, it actually made me wonder if this was done on purpose. With the information that we have available to us, this is a gross injustice to the American consumer.

---

[71] GAO website. FOOD SAFETY: FDA and USDA Should Strengthen Pesticide Residue Monitoring Programs and Further Disclose Monitoring Limitations, October 17, 2014.

Couple this with the science that some pesticides, glyphosate included, are a chelator, meaning that it bonds with some of the minerals in the soil making them less available for uptake from plants. Some studies show that the nutrients are in the soil, but the plants are unable to use them. This is because of the presence of the pesticide and lack of soil biology. To be clear, the pesticide causes a lack of biology, bacterial diversity specifically. Glyphosate can take 9-170 days to break down in the soil. The degradation of glyphosate is relative to many environmental factors such as temperature, water concentration, organic compounds and the microbial base in the soil. Here is the kicker, though: farms that have been sprayed with pesticides have an altered microbial base because of the way they have been managed. So, if pesticides are routinely sprayed, and the soil has not been actively managed *regeneratively,* then it will most likely take longer for it to break down. This means it also has the potential to get into surface and groundwater after a heavy rain, be taken up by the roots of other crops, leaving them open to the development of other crop-specific diseases.[72] In some instances, the residues can actually stay in the soil for up to a year under these sorts of conditions.[73]

Farm Animals, People and Land Symbiosis

So, the deal is that we humans are supposed to live symbiotically with our environments, not destructively. Symbiosis means that there's a mutually beneficial arrangement between the earth, farm animals, plant life, bacteria and fungi in the soil and people. If we treat it well, it will also treat us well. If we use regenerative practices to nurture soil health and overall land management, it

---

[72] Zhao, Q., De Laender, F., & Van den Brink, P. J., Community Composition Modifies Direct and Indirect Effects of Pesticides in Freshwater Food Webs, *Science of The Total Environment*, Volume 739, 2020. https://www.sciencedirect.com/science/article/pii/S0048969720330485?via%3Dihub

[73] *Eco Agriculture Guide. A Complete Systems Approach to Soil Management and Plant Nutrition* https://docs.wixstatic.com/ugd/237db0_3575bcab1c-344b72988e814406aced18.pdf

will provide back a higher quality end plant and animal product that will help our body fight inflammation and oxidative stress and, therefore, disease. The real kicker is that this setup is also best for the environment as well. Sounds like a WIN, WIN, WIN situation to me. All health is local, all the way down to the microbes in the soil.

If we're to manage our farms symbiotically, it must also include regeneration, and part of a regenerative farm could and should also include farm animals. Animals that are raised on organic or regenerative farms are also generally raised on grass or in other natural environments. Remember that we are what we eat but we are also what it eats. If an animal such as a cow, sheep, or bison are raised on grass, their Omega 3 fatty acid content is higher than one that's fed grain over the long term. And even if fed grain only for a short time, the Omega 3 fatty acids diminish with the decrease in grass.[74] Those that are in tune with this will sometimes find food labeling indicating that an end product was "grass-fed" because, at one point, that animal had been raised on grass. I refer you back to the section on food transparency for one of the third-party reviewers that certifies 100% grass-fed animals. The excrement from these animals can also then be used as fertilizer or high nitrogen source for a variety of uses that breaks down much more slowly when managed properly in a regenerative environment rather than synthetic fertilization.

These animals also won't have additional hormones or antibiotics provided to them to grow faster because they're raised in regenerative environments. A study done by Ramatla et al in 2017 showed that between 14.6 to 88% of animal products have antibiotic residues in them depending upon type of antibiotic and kind of animal. Some of these residues showed a concentration well above recommended limits. When I ask my clients if they've had a round of antibiotics recently, I also ask if they buy their meat products from a regenerative farm or

---

[74] Daley, C. A., Abbott, A., Doyle, P. S., Nader, G. A., & Larson, S. A Review of Fatty Acid Profiles and Antioxidant Content in Grass-Fed and Grain-Fed Beef. *Nutrition Journal.* 2010 Mar 10; *9*: 10. https://www.ncbi.nlm.nih.gov/pmc/articles/PMC2846864/

one that has regenerative practices. The reason is because enough of the studies show that these residues are consistently present with the previously referenced study, indicating "The presence of antibiotic residues coupled with multidrug residues in some of the meat samples calls for concern, as this could pose serious public health risks to humans and animals, such as toxicity and resistance development." Veterinary medications are as inevitable as medications are for human beings. We all get sick on occasion. The concern is when the medications are used to increase profit margins with animals raised in less than optimal conditions like CAFOs and then fed to human beings on a large scale. This is where the health risk comes in for humans, animals, and the environment.[75][76]

Since the 1940s, industrialized agriculture has been providing antibiotics and grain to animals to keep them healthy and grow larger, faster. The antibiotics are provided because they're raised in confined quarters where there's greater potential of becoming sick. If there are substantial residues of antibiotics in our food, why would we think there would be less of an impact on human beings? It's known that this is the case by altering the microbiome of people who take antibiotics and/or consume foods with a lot of antibiotic residues. This is one of the many food system contributors to our growing obesity epidemic that will be addressed more in the next chapter.

Estimates are that between 65 to 80% of all antibiotics prescribed in this country are used in animal husbandry practices depending upon the source. Decreased antibiotic susceptibility translates into antibiotic resistance.[77] This

[75] Kaneene, J. B., & Miller, R. Problems Associated With Drug Residues in Beef from Feeds and Therapy. *Reviews in Science & Technology*. 1997 Aug; *16*(2): 694-708. https://pubmed.ncbi.nlm.nih.gov/9501382/

[76] Marshall, B. M., & Levy, S. B. Food Animals and Antimicrobials: Impacts on Human Health. *Clinical Microbiology Review*. 2011 Oct; *24*(4): 718-33. https://pubmed.ncbi.nlm.nih.gov/21976606/

[77] Habboush, Y., & Guzman, N. *Antibiotic Resistance*. StatPearls Publishing; 2022 Jan. https://www.ncbi.nlm.nih.gov/books/NBK513277/https://www.ncbi.nlm.nih.gov/books/NBK513277/

means that when someone gets sick with an infection of an antibiotic-resistant bacteria, there's no antibiotic that can kill this bug. According to the CDC, about 2.8 million people develop antibiotic resistant infections every year. Known drug resistant bacteria include MRSA, VRE, MDR-TB and the newest CRE and are seen in the hospital routinely. While there are major promotions for reductions in unnecessary antibiotic use prescribed by our physicians, the far greater concern is that of our agricultural practices. Additionally, glyphosate, beyond being a registered herbicide and desiccant, is also a registered antibiotic. It is now being reported that pesticide residues are also impacting antibiotic susceptibility in E. coli and salmonella bacteria.[78] We Americans have it coming at us from all different directions in our meat or protein sources as well as on the plants that we eat.

When looking at regenerative farming systems, it must also be considered that anything sustainable over the long term must also have the capacity to regenerate itself on some level. Agricultural inputs in abundance on one part of the farm can be taken and placed in another part of the farm that would help support growth. Regeneration is the process of renewal, restoration, and growth that makes ecosystems resilient to natural fluctuations or events that cause disturbance or damage. When an ecosystem is consistently challenged, rather than providing the amendments necessary to regenerate itself, the natural outcome is that it continues to degrade and can no longer overcome the challenges it faces. The same goes for the human body. If we want our bodies to remain healthy, we must consider what it's being challenged by and how to add back or correct the imbalance.

When the FDA tests for contaminants or pesticides in food, they test for over 200 different compounds. Many of these compounds test within their

---

[78] Kurenbach, B., Marjoshi, D., Amábile-Cuevas, C. F., Ferguson, G. C., Godsoe, W., Gibson, P., & Heinemann, J. A. Sublethal Exposure to Commercial Formulations of the Herbicides Dicamba, 2,4-Dichlorophenoxyacetic Acid, and Glyphosate Cause Changes in Antibiotic Susceptibility in *Escherichia Coli* and *Salmonella Enterica* Serovar Typhimurium. *ASM Journals*, Volume 6, No. 2, March 24, 2015. https://mbio.asm.org/content/6/2/e00009-15

designated limits, but what about those of us who eat a lot of prepackaged food products? What about those folks who eat the Standard American Diet (SAD), high in Omega 6 fats, processed foods, and sugar. Are these folks consuming a much higher amount than this testing accommodates? Some estimate, and it seems reasonable to me, that 75% of the foods found on grocery store shelves have genetically modified food ingredients in them. If this is true, I cannot think of a better reason to start reading food labels to understand more about what we're eating, eat mostly food that doesn't contain a food label, and/or eat more food that comes from a regenerative farm that can be trusted.

Industrialization of Food and Endocrine Disorders

There's certainly a correlative impact of industrialization of food to endocrine disorders in our country including but not necessarily limited to obesity, diabetes, thyroid disorders, and breast cancer. One cannot necessarily say that it has caused the problem but, like most causes of illness, it's multifactorial in nature. No one usually dies directly from obesity or thyroid disorders but they're the underpinning of the rest of our metabolic health, so when our endocrine systems fail us, other health concerns have already crept in. We're just touching on the concerns related to food and agriculture. According to the CDC website, with an increase in obesity comes an increase in the rates of all-cause mortality, diabetes, hypertension, stroke, gallbladder disease, coronary artery disease(-CAD), and many types of cancers.

The Endocrine Society defines an EDC as any "exogenous [non-natural] chemical, or mixture of chemicals, that interferes with any aspect of hormone action." In our food supply, the most likely culprits are persistent organic pollutants including PCBs, pesticides, packaging that uses BPA or any derivatives of this chemical, heavy metals, phthalates also used in packaging (or cosmetics). Some studies show that pesticide residues decrease the good bacteria in animal and human gastrointestinal tracts which allows for the bad bacteria to grow more heartily.[79] BPA and heavy metals significantly alter the gut microbiota causing "dysbiosis" and potentially creating an environment within the GI tract that doesn't support proper digestion and has a potential inflammatory response. Phthalates alter the microbial base, which directly affects microbial metabolites that impact neurological disorders. While there could be much more discussion here, I've provided some references at the end of the book associated with this chapter that can be reviewed if you want to learn more. What I would like you to understand is that none of these chemicals leading to disorders were widely available until the industrialization of food.[80] [81] [82] [83] [84]

I don't have as big a concern about GMOs as much as the pesticide residues and the potential disruptions of our health and our ecosystems. Glyphosate is the number one used herbicide in America promoted under the idea that less

[79] Ackermann, W., Coenen, M., Schrödl, W., Shehata, A. A., & Krüger, M. The Influence of Glyphosate on the Microbiota and Production of Botulinum Neurotoxin During Ruminal Fermentation. *Current Microbiology.* 2015 Mar; *70*(3): 374-82. https://pubmed.ncbi.nlm.nih.gov/25407376/

[80] FDA website, Phthalates in Cosmetics. https://www.fda.gov/cosmetics/cosmetic-ingredients/phthalates

[81] Mnif, W., Hassine, A. I., Bouaziz, A., Bartegi, A., Thomas, O., Roig, B. Effect of Endocrine Disruptor Pesticides: A Review. *International Journal of Environmental Research in Public Health.* 2011 Jun; *8*(6): 2265-2303. https://www.ncbi.nlm.nih.gov/pmc/articles/PMC3138025/

[82] Requena, M., López-Villén, A., Hernández, A. F., Parrón, T., Navarro, Á., & Alarcón, R. Environmental Exposure to Pesticides and Risk of Thyroid Diseases. *Toxicology Letters.* 2019 Oct 15; *315*: 55-63. https://pubmed.ncbi.nlm.nih.gov/31445060/

[83] Samsel, A., & Seneff, S. Glyphosate, Pathways to Modern Diseases III: Manganese, Neurological Diseases, and Associated Pathologies. *Surgical Neurology International.* 2015 Mar 24; *6*: 45. https://www.ncbi.nlm.nih.gov/pmc/articles/PMC4392553/

[84] Seeger, B., Klawonn, F., Nguema Bekale, B., & Steinberg, P. Mixture Effects of Estrogenic Pesticides at the Human Estrogen Receptor α and β. *PLoS One.* 2016 Jan 26; *11*(1): e0147490. https://www.ncbi.nlm.nih.gov/pubmed/26812056

pesticides can be used, but the overall amount every year has gone up and up. As previously stated, 56% of glyphosate use is on genetically engineered crops. This means that the other 44% is on crops that aren't genetically modified or engineered. Recently, the terminology has been changed from GMO to "bioengineered." While the term change may be more descriptive, any name change has the potential to confuse consumers because rarely are these changes covered by the media.

Remember that glyphosate has just recently been added for testing because of the sheer volume of testing that needs to be done to monitor it. This is, of course, backwards thinking, and, as consumers, should scare us, but this may be the least of our worries. Hundreds of pesticides can negatively impact our endocrine system in some capacity or another. Most commonly, they can interfere with natural hormones due to a strong affinity to bind with male or female hormone receptor sites. Some of these, such as DDT, was taken off the market years ago in the United States but, sadly, several countries are still using it and is a part of our international industrialized system.

A recent study reported in the *American Journal of Clinical Nutrition* in February of 2022, "demonstrated that changing to organic food consumption with a Mediterranean Diet high in fruit and vegetables will reduce total pesticide exposure by >90%. This may partially explain the positive health outcomes linked to organic food consumption in observational studies. The study also provided evidence that "increasing fruit and vegetable consumption with conventional foods will substantially increase insecticide and organophosphate exposure."[85] This is important because current public health recommendations for Americans say nothing about pesticide exposure despite a growing body of

---

[85] AJCN on Pesticides in Urine, *The American Journal of Clinical Nutrition*, Volume 115, Issue 2, February 2022, Pages 364–377 https://academic.oup.com/ajcn/article/115/2/364/6412942

evidence that suggests the increase in fruit and vegetable consumption may be offset by the pesticide residues.[86]

This is just one more reason to eat food that's grown regenerative organic and doesn't have a food label on it. So how does someone know if their food has been really raised organically? Those little stickers placed on every single piece of fruit and vegetable in the grocery store will tell you. If the number starts with a 9, it's grown organically. If it starts with an 8 it's genetically modified and if it starts with a 3 or 4 it has been conventionally grown. Conventionally grown doesn't mean pesticide free. Genetically modified most likely means that it has been grown with pesticides. Organically grown means that the only pesticides used are those that are approved by the National Organic Standards Board (NOSB). These are the only statements that can be made across the board because every individual food product will be managed differently.

Additionally, the Environmental Work Group or EWG puts out a list of foods that they revise every year based on their own testing regarding pesticide residues on which of these conventionally raised foods have the highest and lowest levels of pesticide residues. The Dirty Dozen are the fruits and vegetables that have the highest residues and the Clean Fifteen are the fruits and vegetables that would be good choices if one is on a tight budget and not wanting to spend the extra on organic foods. For those who cannot afford to eat organically or regeneratively, the good news is that just washing fruits and vegetables with water can eliminate 70-80% of the pesticide residues on foods. A vinegar or baking soda wash will eliminate up to 98% of pesticides as well as killing most of the bacteria on the produce.

---

[86] Sandoval-Insausti, H., Chiu, Y-H., Wang, Y-X., Hart, J. E., Bhupathiraju, S. N., Mínguez-Alarcón, L., Ding, M., Willett, W. C., Laden, F., & Chavarro, J. E. Intake of Fruits and Vegetables According to Pesticide Residue Status in Relation to All-Cause and Disease-Specific Mortality: Results from Three Prospective Cohort Studies. *Environment International*, Volume 159, 2022. https://reader.elsevier.com/reader/sd/pii/S0160412021006498?token=0AB271EA16326F36886909A66D0472E01FDB0ED34E5F77C541158DE21896CC8E0869B8F2D17C476F549BC1BBF03BD8BD&originRegion=us-east-1&originCreation=20220226204439

Living Downstream of Our Food Supply

It's also important to remember that we all live downstream. If we're cognizant of our agricultural practices, such as fertilization, pesticide use, tending the riparian buffer which supports water retention alongside rivers, we're also aware that when it rains heavily, anything placed on our growing surfaces has the potential to be washed away. The very premise of regenerative agriculture addressed these concerns, but, unfortunately, most of our crops aren't raised this way.

Living in the Midwest, Missouri in particular, with its karst or porous topography, means it goes into our surface and/or groundwater, our lakes and streams, and eventually down to the Gulf of Mexico where there's a large dead zone. This dead zone is roughly between 5,000 - 8,000 square miles in size and the water contains less than 2 ppb or parts per billion of dissolved oxygen, essentially deeming it "dead." For perspective, aerobic or oxygen-loving bacteria cannot maintain life below 6 ppb. This lack of oxygen is a direct reflection of the amount of nutrients, mainly nitrogen and phosphorus, that aren't being retained on farms, lawns, and effluent from wastewater treatment plants that are making their way down to the Gulf of Mexico. The lion's share of this comes from the farming operations in the Mississippi River Basin. This has a direct impact on aquatic life as the increase in fertilization encourages algae growth which throws the ecosystem out of balance and diminishes the oxygen content of the water. This is known as eutrophication. This eutrophication has been shown to reduce biomass and biodiversity. Fish cannot live in a part of the ocean that doesn't have oxygen in it. Our largest dead zone is the Gulf of Mexico, but sadly there are many all over the world.

This concept of living downstream applies to any residues of the agricultural process. CAFOs are notorious for contaminating groundwater with Escherichia coli or E. coli in particular, a potentially deadly bacteria. Here in Missouri, one can often see cattle wading in the local streams which has a direct impact on what's colonized in the water. Missouri also has more than 400,000 private wells in the state. Studies done in the 1990s indicated that many people have wells that are at risk for Escherichia coli and nitrates from improper placement, maintenance, or testing of their wells.[87] Because of the porous nature of the land in Missouri, as well as the restrictions that have been lifted on CAFOs, there will continue to be E. coli and nitrate contamination in our local water due to improper management of manure associated with these operations.

While not the only source of these contaminants, they're the major source of them. Another source of agricultural nitrates would be inorganic fertilizers. In the spring every year, the nitrate levels in groundwater increase because of the runoff of these fertilizers.[88]

Nitrates have an additional impact on the thyroid as well as raising cancer rates. According to 2010 Article by Ward et al. entitled, "Nitrate intake and the risk of thyroid cancer and thyroid disease" nitrates inhibit thyroid uptake of iodide by binding to the sodium-iodide symporter on the surface of thyroid follicles.[89] This increases Thyroid Stimulating Hormone (TSH) because it reduces the amount of T3 and T4 or thyroid hormones in the blood. This is another good reason to have an RO filtration system in your house if you have a well where there's also a CAFO close by when you or someone in your family struggles with thyroid concerns. Guess what also contains lots of nitrates? Highly processed meat products like hot dogs, sausages, and bacon. Nitrates help to preserve the pretty pink color in processed meats. If we aren't careful, nitrates are in our water and on our plates. If you want to find out more about what's in your well water, local health departments have the capability of testing wells for contaminants

---

[87] CDC website. https://www.cdc.gov/healthywater/drinking/private/wells/testing.html

[88] Ward, M. H. Too Much of a Good Thing? Nitrate from Nitrogen Fertilizers and Cancer. *Review of Environmental Health.* 2009 Oct-Dec; *24*(4):357-363 https://www.ncbi.nlm.nih.gov/pmc/articles/PMC3068045/

[89] Ward, M. H., Kilfoy, B. A., Weyer, P.J., Anderson, K. E., Folsom, A. R., & Cerhan, J. R. Nitrate Intake and the Risk of Thyroid Cancer and Thyroid Disease. *Epidemiology.* 2010 May;*21*(3):https://www.ncbi.nlm.nih.gov/pmc/articles/PMC2879161/#:~:text=Ingested%20nitrate%20inhibits%20thyroid%20uptake,thyroid%20stimulating%20hormone%20(TSH).

How Does This Translate Into Health Outcomes?

If we're fortunate, every day, we have the opportunity to get up in the morning, go to work, eat, exercise, go to sleep, get up, and do it again the next day. Our bodies are always under some degree of stress. If we eat right, exercise, and cope well, we provide our bodies with the substrate or tools to manage that stress, including what's provided to our bodies in the food we eat and the water we drink. What causes ill health? Our ill health is ultimately caused by our bodies not having support for the systems that keep us healthy or being overburdened and unable to handle the additional stress load. I'll be explaining a little more about this in the next chapter.

Just remember, food is agriculture. Agriculture is food. When we eat too much food from the conventional agricultural system, we add an additional stress to our body systems very similar to what's inflicted on the earth by this kind of agriculture. The symbiosis that occurs when we treat the earth well, by nurturing it regeneratively, also supports our own health. The same anaerobic bacteria that can make plants sick can make people sick as well. The runoff from improperly managed dirt gets into the groundwater and can influence our health outcomes. When we treat the earth well, it returns a higher-quality food product with higher levels of those inflammation- and oxidative-stress-fighting phytochemicals, meat products that are higher in anti-inflammatory Omega 3 fatty acids, no antibiotic, bacterial, nitrogenous or pesticide residues to disrupt our microbiome or endocrine system. We then provide our bodies the opportunity to rest and heal itself without the additional stressors associated with conventionally raised food.

Does this mean that if you switch over to what's essentially deemed clean eating, you'll feel immediately better? Many do. There are also a significant percentage of people whose diets are so poor that initially they need to detox, feel sicker first, before they start feeling better. To those people, I suggest making a slow change and hanging there for the long haul. If we all ate better, we would at least see lower rates of the underlying disease processes that plague our country such as thyroid disorders, obesity, heart disease, and diabetes. There will be more on these disease rates in the next chapter.

Many people also lament about the expense of food that's raised properly. To them I usually tell them to start a garden. While this sounds perhaps flippant, once they've put the effort into understanding what it takes for a farmer to have food readily available at a farmers' market or otherwise, they become grateful quite quickly that it only costs them what it does. Gratitude changes attitude. We Americans will spend tens of thousands of dollars on a vehicle but complain about the expense of grass-fed organic ground beef at $10.00 a pound. A shift in the paradigm must occur for folks to see that a little up-front investment in their health, by supporting regenerative farmers, could save them thousands of dollars and perhaps provide many additional, healthy years on the planet in the long run. I, for one, want to be around to enjoy my grandchildren and not from a wheelchair. It's a quality-of-life issue.

This paradigm shift needs to occur early in life. Children from a young age should be taught about food and agriculture so there's a literacy around these very fundamental supports of life. I notice that many times, when I start having a conversation with people who don't understand that our food system in America is quite broken, they glaze over pretty quickly. It's not that they're not incapable of understanding but, unless one has had some exposure to the issues and terminology, it seems quite overwhelming and hopeless. People need to know what our current system is and how the system became broken so that we know what we, as individuals, can do to help ourselves. Hopefully, it has been made clearer in the preceding pages. We need to not be afraid to get our hands dirty in the soil. We need to teach our children how to grow food and impress upon them the importance of teaching their children how to grow food, handing down this information from generation to generation.

While it would be great if McDonald's provided regenerative grass-fed beef, locally sourced salad greens, a specialty pickle product from the farm down the street that grows cucumbers, and local kombucha on tap, I don't believe this will ever be cost worthy. Local restaurants could purposefully engage these local food endeavors and be supported by the local community spending food dollars at their establishment so they can persevere. The former would be a pipe dream that would ultimately send the price of a burger to $10 instead of the dollar menu and potentially put them out of business. This wouldn't make me sad. This is the right map, however, the roadmap of regenerative food and agriculture, from which to plan our health journey.

7.
The Broken Steering Wheel

I would be remiss in my duties as a dietitian if I didn't bring to light a factor that's separate from our food systems but also influences our health dramatically. The steering wheel of our health is our medical system. If we could empower ourselves by understanding more about how it functions and if it weren't broken as well, we would be able to turn the vehicle in whatever direction that we decided, working in cooperation with our physicians. Health should be cooperatively decided regarding what's needed to prevent or improve a health circumstance. This isn't what happens most often in conventional medicine, however.

The unfortunate reality is that insurance dictates which doctor you can see, what services are covered, and what medicines you can take. Have you ever had a change in insurance and then had to change doctors and medications? How many times have you been told what service you could have or what prescription for what illness was allowed? This usually means that any step outside of the system discourages service coverage and one will have to pay for that service or medication out of pocket or at least more for the service.

To take it one step further, insurance coverage is dictated on a large scale by the government. The coverage for Medicare and Medicaid is governed by The Centers for Medicaid and Medicare Coverage (CMS) which is under the umbrella of the Department of Health and Human Services (DHHS). This includes coverage for over 58 million people across the United States. They provide the guidelines for what will be covered for a given service. Included in the references are the guidelines for Medicare Coverage Part A and B. Coverage providers are told this from the start.[90] If one goes online, a lot of energy from these organizations is put forth to encourage medication compliance and we'll talk about medication usage in the coming pages. The greatest most recent example of how this works would have been with the COVID crisis. If a physician did some research and felt that a medication was outside of what the government allows and they wanted to prescribe it to one of their patients, it wouldn't be covered by insurance and they could have lost their license. Why? Because it wasn't approved by the CDC or FDA, both federal agencies, for this use. Whether one believes this is the best choice or not is actually not the point. The point is that the physician wasn't allowed to medically make what they thought was the best decision for their patient.

On the whole, our current conventional medical system practices reactive medical care and reductionist medicine. Reactive medical care is essentially providing medical care AFTER something goes wrong, after we've lost control of our vehicles and driven off the cliff, rather than supporting preventative health. And when medical care is provided, it works off the assumption that a medical problem can be separated into smaller more simple parts rather than looking at it from the systems biology standpoint. Systems biology is the approach to biomedical research that looks at the larger picture. It takes into consideration that the body is one large system rather than breaking it down into smaller pieces.

Let me give a simple example to explain this further. A patient goes to the doctor's office because they've had persistent reflux symptoms for the last several weeks that won't go away. The physician does a short physical exam, takes blood pressure, weighs the patients, asks a few questions and then prescribes a Proton Pump Inhibitor (PPI) for reflux symptoms and sends them home to fill the prescription and feel better. The patient is 30 pounds overweight after gaining 30 pounds in the last two years, doesn't exercise, and eats fast food or sit-down restaurant food for at least half of the meals consumed. At no point during this

---

[90] Medicare Benefits, This official government booklet has important information about the items and services Original Medicare covers, 2022. https://www.medicare.gov/Pubs/pdf/10116-your-medicare-benefits.pdf

interaction does the physician discuss losing weight, changing diet, or initiating an exercise program. This person then continues to take the PPI for years because the symptoms never really go away. They're just masked until something else goes wrong because the underlying cause of the problem was never addressed.

PPIs are some of the most prescribed medicines in America. They can be identified by the generic name that ends in "-prazole" such as omeprazole and pantoprazole. Some of the brand names would be Prilosec, Prevacid, and Nexium. They're not designed to be taken long term because their mechanism of action is to decrease stomach acid and, therefore, decrease the symptoms of reflux, and they're very effective in doing this. Patients do, in fact, feel better, which can be a deterrent to motivate any other behavior changes. They're not designed to be taken long term however because decreasing stomach acid or pH has side effects. Stomach acid is essential for the absorption of minerals and micronutrients as well as keeping bacterial balance in the GI tract and keeping the pH low enough to support detoxification systems in the body.

At this point, there's enough scientific literature to support the fact that PPIs, if used long term, can promote B12 deficiency, low magnesium levels, altered calcium metabolism, and anemia.[91] Functionally, what goes along with this is increased rates of bone fractures, increased rates of dementia, and potential clostridium difficile or C diff infections from dysbiosis in the GI tract. C diff is a particularly nasty gut bacteria referenced previously that can cause loose water diarrhea for days or weeks at time.

Does any of this sound like fun? These are very real situations that we see in the hospital every day because some people are left on these medications for decades. Yes, decades. Preventative medical care and systems biology approach would have avoided additional possible side effects from one more medication over the long term. The interaction in the office should have gone more like this.

---

[91] Maes, M. L., Fixen, D. R., & Linnebur, S. A. Adverse Effects of Proton-Pump Inhibitor Use in Older Adults: A Review of the Evidence. *Therapeutic Advances in Drug Safety*. 2017 Sep; *8*(9): 273-297. https://www.ncbi.nlm.nih.gov/pmc/articles/PMC5557164/

> "I understand that you aren't feeling well Mr./Mrs. So and So, but I also see here from your medical records that over the past two years you have gained 30 pounds and your blood pressure is up slightly. Tell me about this. What do you think has affected this?"

After listening and understanding the patient's circumstance.

> "It sounds as though life has been a bit stressful for you and your family. I'm happy to prescribe you some medication over the short term but I would also like you to look at implementing a diet and exercise program because ultimately that will help the problem more holistically over the long term. You'll need to stop eating out so much and lose some weight, which will help to reduce symptoms as well as take fried foods entirely out of your diet. Would you like to try this on your own or would you like a referral to a dietitian and an exercise specialist to put together programs with you?"

When prescribing medicine, without a mention of diet and exercise we aren't addressing the root cause or the disrupted biological system that's creating the problem to begin with. PPIs in particular have the capacity to create major disruptions in the multiple biological systems including the Gastrointestinal Tract (microbiome, C. diff), Orthopedic (bone fracture), Neurological Systems (dementia) and Hematological Systems (anemia) mentioned previously. But wait; it's just a little reflux medication. Most Americans don't know enough to even question the approach.

Over Medicated and Under Healed

We are living longer than ever before on more medication than ever before. Our disease rates are on the rise as is our medication usage. And what comes with this are the disruptions that are caused within different biological systems that cannot heal themselves while on these medications and with suboptimal nutrition. Mortality statistics on the CDC site for 2019 show that the top nine out of ten causes of death are all influenced by nutrition. The 2020 changes are in the parentheses to the right.

Heart Disease - 659,041 - (Up 4.1%)

Cancer - 599,601- (Down 1.4%)

Accidents - 173,040- (Up 16.8%)

Chronic Lower Respiratory Illness -156,979 (Down 4.7%)

Stroke -150,005 (Up 4.9%)

Alzheimer's -121,499 (Up 8.7%)

Diabetes - 87,647 (Up 14.8%)

Influenza and Pneumonia - 51,565 (Up 5.7%)

Kidney Disease - 49,595 (Unchanged)

Self-Harm/Suicide - 47,511- (dropped from list as COVID was added in 2020)[92]

The only mortality statistic that's not directly influenced by nutrition is accidental deaths. From these numbers, only 8.2% of deaths out of 2,096,671 deaths in 2019 weren't influenced by nutrition. This doesn't account for the underlying causes of these illnesses including hypertension, obesity, autoimmunity, or thyroid dysfunction which are all also directly influenced by nutrition and very much on the rise as well. One could also argue that there's statistical information that COVID deaths could have been also mitigated by adequate vitamin D stores which could also be considered a nutrition-related death[93]. It should addi-

---

[92] Sherry, L., Murphy, B. S., Kenneth, D., Kochanek, M. A., & Jiaquan, Xu, & Arias, E. Mortality 2020, CDC. https://www.cdc.gov/nchs/data/databriefs/db427.pdf

[93] Borsche, L., Glauner, B., & von Mendel, J. COVID-19 Mortality Risk Correlates Inversely with Vitamin D3 Status, and a Mortality Rate Close to Zero Could Theoretically Be Achieved at 50 ng/mL 25(OH)D3: Results of a Systematic Review and Meta-Analysis. *Nutrients*. 2021 Oct 14; *13*(10): 3596. https://www.ncbi.nlm.nih.gov/pmc/articles/PMC8541492/

tionally noted that the mortality associated with COVID was highest in people with comorbidities.[94] This realistically explains any drops on the above chart.

> The CDC published, "From 2019 to 2020, age-adjusted death rates increased for 6 of 10 leading causes of death and decreased for 2. The rate increased 4.1% for heart disease (from 161.5 in 2019 to 168.2 in 2020), 16.8% for unintentional injuries (49.3 to 57.6), 4.9% for stroke (37.0 to 38.8), 8.7% for Alzheimer's disease (29.8 to 32.4), 14.8% for diabetes (21.6 to 24.8), and 5.7% for influenza and pneumonia (12.3 to 13.0). Rates decreased 1.4% for cancer (146.2 to 144.1) and 4.7% for chronic lower respiratory diseases (38.2 to 36.4). The rate for kidney disease remained unchanged."

Obesity wasn't even recognized by the American Medical Association (AMA) as a disease until 2013. Being overweight isn't necessarily unhealthy, in and of itself, but the opportunity to diagnose obesity now meant that medical care associated with it could be covered by insurance and the diagnosis of obesity perhaps needed a treatment plan. To be clear, weight loss consultation prior to this time and, subsequently, for a long time after, wasn't covered by insurance for this reason. Although it's not thought of as a condition that one dies from, it contributes directly to the top 9 out of 10 reasons people die in America. The rates of obesity in the last 30 years have skyrocketed. Currently, more than 1 out of 3 people in America are overweight, 2 in 5 adults are obese and 1 in 11 adults have severe obesity.[95] Statistically, the earlier in life that one is overweight the

---

[94] Djaharuddin, I., Munawwarah, S., Nurulita, A., Ilyas, M., Tabri, N. A., & Lihawa, N. Comorbidities and Mortality in COVID-19 Patients. *Gaceta Sanitaria* 2021; *35* Suppl 2: S530-S532. https://pubmed.ncbi.nlm.nih.gov/34929892/

[95] NIH website, Obesity Stats. https://www.niddk.nih.gov/health-information/health-statistics/overweight-obesity#trends

more likely they are to become overweight or obese as an adolescent or adult. Further, the standards for being overweight or obese have not changed over the years. People really are larger.

What comes with obesity is a host of other concerns that come under the umbrellas of metabolic syndrome or syndrome X. Notice that this isn't on the top ten list either. It's because it's a subset of symptoms including high blood pressure, high blood sugar, unhealthy cholesterol levels, and abdominal adiposity. As previously mentioned, being overweight isn't necessarily unhealthy; it's when the rest of these concerns go unnoticed that they start creating long-term side effects. Insulin resistance is the precursor of high blood sugars and because one can be insulin resistant or prediabetic without high blood sugars, it goes unnoticed. If you're concerned about prediabetes, insulin resistance, or metabolic syndrome, I would refer you to a new book called *Your Plate is Your Fate* by a cohort of mine, Dr. Steve Hughlett. He cuts to the chase about dietary guidelines as well as recommendations for addressing this from the nutrition standpoint that I fully endorse. He advocates for lower carbohydrate, higher vegetable intakes that would benefit us all.

Hopefully, it has become easier to see that this issue isn't just calories in vs. calories out. It's also an issue of antibiotic and pesticide residues, nitrates, PFAS, and BPA in our food supply. When our microbiomes are disrupted, putting people on low-calorie diets and expecting them to lose weight has only limited effectiveness. This is the very reason why I became passionate about addressing the issues within our food systems. The youngest child I saw in the hospital with obesity and insulin resistance, a precursor to diabetes, was less than 3-years-old. That was over a decade and a half ago. We aren't heading in the right direction.

Thyroid dysregulation is perhaps one of the more confusing endocrine concerns that needs more research. Thirty years ago, it used to be that slender people with slightly bulging eyes had hyperthyroidism or Graves' disease and folks that tended to be overweight had hypothyroidism. One could almost tell by looking at the physical characteristics of the individual because it played out quite directly, metabolically, which impacted physical appearance. This isn't even close to the case anymore. Underweight or people with a healthy BMI are being diagnosed with sluggish thyroid and overweight folks are being diagnosed with overactive thyroids or both.

According to a research paper in *Advances in Therapy* in 2019, "Environmental iodine deficiency is the most common cause of thyroid disorders, including hypothyroidism, worldwide, while in areas of iodine sufficiency, the most common cause of primary hypothyroidism is autoimmune thyroiditis (Hashimoto's disease)."[96] It's estimated that 5% of the population struggles with some form of thyroid disorder and that another 5% goes undiagnosed. Why does this matter? Thyroid disorders contribute to goiter, heart problems, mental health issues, peripheral neuropathy, and for women of child-bearing age, infertility and birth defects. And as previously mentioned there's quite a bit going on with our food system that impacts our thyroid as well. Is it iodine deficiency or competition for absorption? Additionally, in functional nutrition, any autoimmune disorder has its roots in a leaky gut and foreign material getting into the bloodstream that then impacts a given organ. Thyroid disorders can be classified as either endocrine or autoimmune depending upon the cause. In this case, the thyroid and autoimmunity didn't make the top 10 but, like obesity, the impact is far-reaching and part of an increasingly complicated medical picture for many people. Rarely would there be a diagnosis of just thyroid dysfunction.

Most people are being diagnosed with more than two disease processes or what are called comorbidities at the same time, forcing physicians to decide what to focus on based on the most immediate need. Comorbidities have been shown to be associated with adverse health outcomes, poor quality of life, and increased mortality for this reason. "Individuals with comorbidities account for over 60% of total health care expenditures and 98% of Medicare expenditures."[97]

---

[96] Chiovato, L., Magri, F., & Carlé, A. Hypothyroidism in Context: Where We've Been and Where We're Going. *Advances in Therapy.* 2019 Sep; *36*(Suppl 2): 47-58. https://www.ncbi.nlm.nih.gov/pmc/articles/PMC6822815/

[97] Van Cleave, J. H., Trotta, R.L., Lysaght, S., Steis, M. R., Lorenz, R. A., Naylor, M. D. Comorbidities in the Context of Care Transitions. *Advances in Nursing Science.*

As Americans, if born in 2020, we're currently projected to live, on average, to 77. This is down 1.8 years from 2019 mostly attributed to COVID.

If we're fortunate to live until 77, it's also likely to be on multiple medications or in the context of something called polypharmacy. Polypharmacy is the use of more than one medication, most commonly defined as five or more, however. The concern with polypharmacy is that the more medications one takes, the more likely that drug/drug interactions as well as drug/nutrient interactions can occur. More than half of the country takes four or more medications and many of us are also taking vitamins and supplements along with these medications.[98]

According to a different *Consumer Reports* article[99],1.3 million people went to U.S. emergency rooms due to adverse drug effects in 2014, and about 124,000 died from those events. That's 9.5% of people who had reactions! The total number of prescriptions filled in 1997 was close to 2.5 billion. In 2016, it was close to 4.5 billion with a population increase of only 23%. A 2018 survey from the Council of Responsible Nutrition[100] indicated that 75% of Americans are also taking supplements which represents a 10% increase in the last 10 years. So, the next time one of those TV commercials comes on that promotes a medication to fix a single problem, then toward the second half starts rattling off all the potential side effects, take it quite seriously. We've become a pill-popping society with very little consideration for the side effects of taking these medications.

2013 Apr-Jun; *36*(2). https://www.ncbi.nlm.nih.gov/pmc/articles/PMC4485407/

[98] Masnoon, N., Shakib, S., Kalisch-Ellett, L., & Caughey, G. E. What Is Polypharmacy? A Systematic Review of Definitions. *BMC Geriatrics*. 2017 Oct 10; *17*(1): 230. https://www.ncbi.nlm.nih.gov/pmc/articles/PMC5635569/

[99] Carr, T. Too Many Meds: America's love Affair with Prescription Medication , *Consumer Reports*, August 2017.https://www.consumerreports.org/prescription-drugs/too-many-meds-americas-love-affair-with-prescription-medication/

[100] Council on Responsible Nutrition website.. https://www.crnusa.org/2018ConsumerSurvey#:·:text=According%20to%20the%202018%20survey,%E2%80%9334%20(69%20percent).&text=Data%20show%20that%2083%20percent,percentage%20points%20from%20last%20year.

The top 12 prescriptions, ranked in order from most prescribed to least in 2020 according to ClinCalc Database are: Atorvastatin (cholesterol), Levothyroxine (low thyroid), Metformin (Type 2 Diabetes), Lisinopril (high blood pressure), Amlodipine (blood pressure), Metoprolol (blood pressure), Albuterol (rescue inhaler), Omeprazole (reflux), Losartan (blood pressure), simvastatin (cholesterol), Gabapentin (peripheral neuropathy, nerve pain), Hydrochlorothiazide (diuretic), Sertraline HCL (depression, PTSD), and Simvastatin (cholesterol).[101] These represent between 114 million to almost 44 million prescriptions per medication per year and every one of them could be reduced by diet and exercise.

Diet and exercise influences weight, cardiovascular health, and the micro-biome or your gut, which also, in turn, influence blood pressure, pain response, psychological health, thyroid, cholesterol levels, detoxification systems, reflux, and kidney and lung health. However, it doesn't mean that there are no situations where these medications are necessary but if they're being prescribed long term without prescriptions for diet and exercise, it's a set-up for long-term ill health because the root cause is never addressed. At a minimum, it should come with a politely suggested trip to the farmers' market, a number of different types of vegetables to try, new recipes for the week, and to go out for a long, daily walk. Without this additional prescription, our physicians are doing us, their patients, an enormous disservice.

It's estimated that over 20% of hospitalized patients are malnourished before they come to the hospital for medical care, with Americans over the age of 70 being at highest risk.[102] Being malnourished is also associated with less positive medical outcomes as well as longer hospital stays. These are also the folks who

[101] Top Prescribed Meds in 2020, ClinCalc Database. https://clincalc.com/DrugStats/Top300Drugs.aspx

[102] Kang, M. C. et al. Korean Society for Parenteral and Enteral Nutrition (KSPEN) Clinical Research Groups. Prevalence of Malnutrition in Hospitalized Patients: a Multicenter Cross-sectional Study. *Journal of Korean Medical Science.* 2018 Jan 8; *33*(2): e10. https://www.ncbi.nlm.nih.gov/pmc/articles/PMC5729651

are taking more medications. What goes right along with taking medications and the potential for drug/drug interactions is the potential for drug/nutrient interactions. Many of the medications most prescribed in the hospital are on the top 12 list and have substantial drug nutrient medication reactions that can potentially contribute to the further degeneration of our health. These drug/nutrient interactions either increase the need for certain nutrients or alter the metabolism of the nutrients in some way. These interactions can also be either positive or negative regarding the absorption of the drug depending upon the influence of food. This is especially true if taken daily as they're prescribed. The following medications of the top 12 have identified drug/nutrient interactions:

Statins (cholesterol lowering medications) - Co Q10, mitochondrial health, significant increased risk for diabetes, grapefruit
Antibiotics - B vitamins and disruptions of the microbiome
Levothyroxine- Calcium and Iron
Metformin- B12
Blood Pressure medications - B vitamins, grapefruit
PPI - Magnesium, Calcium, Iron, B12
Diuretics - B vitamins, electrolytes, Calcium, magnesium and zinc
Sertraline- nausea, diarrhea, weight gain[103]

Also, as a part of the overall nutrition evaluation, dietitians look for the physical signs of nutritional deficiency or a Nutrition Focused Physical Exams (NFPE). These exams are targeted at looking specifically for micronutrient deficiencies in the human body, and you might be surprised how many are found. It's especially prevalent in the older segments of the population who are sometimes hospitalized with over 10 medications and haven't been eating well for a long while. Supplementation to correct the deficiencies then becomes part of the Medical Nutrition Therapy (MNT) for these patients. Patients who show nutrient deficiencies cannot truly start the healing process until the deficiency is

---

[103] ELO Smart Nutrition website https://www.elo.health/articles/surprising-drug-nutrient-interactions/

addressed and perhaps corrected. What's not known is to what degree medications are influencing these micronutrient deficiencies, but they're certainly one more layer of concern when it comes to the health of Americans.

What we do know is that too much medication along with the Standard American Diet (SAD) can contribute to disruptions in the microbiome. As stated before, the rates of all gastrointestinal, autoimmune, and neurodegenerative related disorders are on the rise and overmedication could be part of the reason for this. Our GI tracts are essentially the gateway to the rest of our health.

Supplementation Not Regulated as Medicine

Let's talk about supplement regulation for a minute. While technically under the umbrella of the Federal Drug Administration (FDA) in the United States, the estimated $133 billion global supplement industry is one of the few industries that regulates itself in our country. According to a survey from the Council on Responsible Nutrition, 75% of Americans take supplements.[104] There are an estimate 23,000 ER visits per year due to interactions with supplements[105], but a supplement only gets removed from the market if it's reported and proven to have caused a health concern from consumers, other supplement companies, or other concerned citizens.[106] The process for making it to market is significantly less cumbersome than over-the-counter medications or prescription medications. Supplement companies are required to submit evidence that their products are safe and don't contain impurities or provide the consumer misleading

---

[104] Grebow, J. 75% of Americans Take Dietary Supplements, Latest CRN Survey Finds, *Nutritional Outlook*, October 19, 2018. http://www.nutritionaloutlook.com/trends-business/75-americans-take-dietary-supplements-latest-crn-survey-finds

[105] Geller, A. I., Shehab, N., Weidle, N. J., Lovegrove, M. C., Wolpert, B. J., Timbo, B. B., Mozersky, R. P., & Budnitz, D. S. Emergency Department Visits for Adverse Events Related to Dietary Supplements. *New England Journal of Medicine*. 2015 Oct 15; *373*(16) https://pubmed.ncbi.nlm.nih.gov/26465986/

[106] FDA website, Supplements. https://www.fda.gov/food/dietary-supplements

marketing. They're only required to submit safety data for new ingredients on the market, and the FDA can only take action after a product has been misbranded or adulterated after it's already on the market. Sounds a bit backwards for such a large industry.

This is why I only recommend supplements that have been third-party reviewed, have a proven track record from arbitrary third-party batch testing, return phone calls when requested, and have no history of tainted supplements. Any consumer can access a variety of third-party supplement testing through places like Consumer Labs. If you're seriously considering taking supplements, please take the time to educate yourself on what supplement you should be taking. Check their websites for batch testing results. Some manufacturers that perform this batch testing will post it on their sites. If they don't have results available, call the manufacturer and ask. If they don't return the call, don't buy the supplement.

One of the most prescribed supplements on the market (7.9% of the total market) are fish oil/ Omega 3/DHA, EPA fatty acids.[107] They're so prominent in the market because they're so important for our health impacting cardiovascular disease, dyslipidemia in diabetes, mental health, autoimmunity, thyroid, arthritis, asthma, or essentially any disease process associated with inflammation.[108] [109]

[107] National Center for Complementary and Integrative Health, NIH on Supplements. https://www.nccih.nih.gov/health/using-dietary-supplements-wisely

[108] Balk, E. M., Adams, G. P., Langberg, V., Halladay, C., Chung, M., Lin, L., Robertson, S., Yip, A., Steele, D., Smith, B. T., Lau, J., Lichtenstein, A. H., & Trikalinos, T. A. Omega-3 Fatty Acids and Cardiovascular Disease: An Updated Systematic Review. *Evidence Report: Technology Assessment* 2016 Aug;(223):1-1252. https://pubmed.ncbi.nlm.nih.gov/30307737/

[109] Friedberg, C. E., Janssen, M. J., Heine, R. J., & Grobbee, D. E. Fish Oil and Glycemic Control in Diabetes. A Meta-Analysis. *Diabetes Care.* 1998 Apr; *21*(4): 494-500. https://pubmed.ncbi.nlm.nih.gov/9571330/

[110]Many studies have been done that indicated over half of the supplements don't meet the claims that they put on the label for amounts of EPA/DHA and up to one quarter don't meet industry standards for peroxidase values, a measure of whether the supplements were oxidized or not.[111] Oxidation essentially renders the supplement ineffective for its likely intended purpose and/or potentially even harmful.[112] And this is just one supplement example in a sea of hundreds of thousands of examples. Here's the deal, though. We consume fewer Omega-3 fatty acids in our diet now, because of an industrialized food system. If it shifted back would we need them any longer? I don't think anyone knows the answer to this but it's certainly worth some consideration to eat some additional grass-fed meats.

As an industrialized country, one would expect objectively that we should be living long healthy lives. The unfortunate truth is that the next generation of children won't be living longer than the current aging generation. We're living longer currently but sicker than ever before. And we should be asking ourselves why? The supplements industry would have us believing that taking their supplements would have us living longer, but, to date, I'm unaware of any literature that provides statistical evidence that this is true.

Dr. Bruce Ames and his cohorts have come up with some ideas about why we aren't living longer. Dr. Ames is a Senior Scientist at Children's Hospital Oakland

---

[110] Montori, V. M., Farmer, A., Wollan, P. C., & Dinneen, S. F. Fish Oil Supplementation in Type 2 Diabetes: A Quantitative Systematic Review. *Diabetes Care*. 2000 Sep; *23*(9):1407-15. https://pubmed.ncbi.nlm.nih.gov/10977042/?from_term=quality+fish+oil+supplements&from_page=6&from_pos=2

[111] Ritter, J. C., Budge, S. M., & Jovica, F. Quality Analysis of Commercial Fish Oil Preparations. *Journal of the Science of Food and Agriculture*. 2013 Jun; *93*(8): 1935-9. https://pubmed.ncbi.nlm.nih.gov/23255124/?from_term=quality+fish+oil+supplements&from_page=3&from_pos=1

[112] Mason, R. P., & Sherratt, S. C. R. Omega-3 Fatty Acid Fish Oil Dietary Supplements Contain Saturated Fats and Oxidized Lipids That May Interfere With Their Intended Biological Benefits. *Biochemical Biophysical Research Communication*. 2017 Jan 29; *483*(1): 425-429. https://pubmed.ncbi.nlm.nih.gov/28011269/?from_term=oxidized+fish+oil+&from_pos=1

Research Institute (CHORI), Director of their Nutrition & Metabolism Center, and a Professor Emeritus of Biochemistry and Molecular Biology, University of California, Berkeley. His publications promote the understanding that subclinical nutritional deficiencies (deficiency that wouldn't be noted on a physical exam necessarily unless nutrient focused) contribute to overall morbidity or illness and that low micronutrient intakes are accelerating our disease process. During periods of low nutrient intakes, much like what we see with intakes of our industrialized food system, our bodies "triage" for short-term survival over longevity.[113] Low micronutrient intakes can be seen in diets that consume high amounts of refined foods with lots of sugar, otherwise known as junk food.

How do we ensure that we aren't triaging nutrients? Keep ourselves as healthy as possible. Eat foods grown or raised regeneratively that don't have labels and keep our microbiome healthy. The list of supportive information for this theory shows how different nutrient deficiencies are related to a variety of diseases of aging. These associations, certainly not allowed on any food label, include selenium and congestive heart failure (CHF), Vitamin K1 and K2 with lower all cause cancer and cardiovascular disease (CVD) mortality, vitamin D and all-cause mortality and cancer.[114] [115]The cool thing about vitamin D is that many people can raise levels just by getting outside in the garden and getting some sun for 20 minutes during the middle of the day.

Triage theory also suggests that some "nutrients" have not necessarily been viewed as essential. In nutritional terms, essential means that one would have

---

[113] Ames, B. Triage Theory. http://www.bruceames.org/Triage.pdf

[114] McCann, J. C., & Ames, B. N. Vitamin K, an Example of Triage Theory: Is Micronutrient Inadequacy Linked to Diseases of Aging? *American Journal of Clinical Nutrition.* 2009 Oct; *90*(4): 889-907. https://pubmed.ncbi.nlm.nih.gov/19692494/

[115] Bomer, N., Grote Beverborg, N., Hoes, M. F., Streng, K. W., Vermeer, M., Dokter, M. M., Ijmker, J., Anker, S. D., Cleland, J. G. F., Hillege, H. L., Lang, C. C., Ng, L. L., Samani, N. J., Tromp, J., van Veldhuisen, D. J., Touw, D. J., Voors, A. A., & van der Meer, P. Selenium and Outcome in Heart Failure. European Journal of Heart Failure. 2020 Aug; *22*(8): 1415-1423. https://pubmed.ncbi.nlm.nih.gov/31808274/

to consume them in order to have them available for your body to assimilate, as your body doesn't manufacture them on its own. These other "nutrients" fall in the category of phytochemicals or components of food associated with the natural color of foods. Remember the discussion in the last chapter about these compounds being higher in plants grown in regenerated soil? Phytochemical research is really just in its infancy regarding our understanding of the benefits that they provide in our bodies and whether they could possibly be classified as true, essential nutrients or not. Regardless, many are antioxidants, which help our bodies process oxidative stress, while others provide anti-inflammatory benefits. The important thing here is to eat your colors from real food to capitalize on the value that they provide.

Phytochemicals can now be supplemented as well. But again, there really is no substitution for eating right. Remember that these are also the components of food that are lower in fruits, vegetables, and grains that aren't raised regeneratively or, at least, organically raised. Also remember that, as long as our bodies are working properly, we assimilate all components of food much more efficiently when in its original form. Therefore, food would be the preferred method of delivery and, since the foods that are high in phytochemicals don't come with a food label, a good understanding of how to identify and locate regeneratively raised foods around the area that you live in, continues to be an essential part of the paradigm shift.

Stress and Nutrition

Another important aspect of managing health that doesn't get addressed routinely is stress. As previously mentioned, we live in a society of convenience whereby the emphasis has been placed on doing more with less and squeezing every last bit into our already packed full lives.

This essentially keeps us in a state of fight or flight or engaging the sympathetic nervous system. This part of our nervous system has been instrumental in keeping us alive since the beginning of time as it's that system that revs up our heart rate and gets us ready to fight the charge of an oncoming elephant. Fortunately, we no longer have these sorts of assaults in our modern day lives, yet a large segment of society continually engages in the sympathetic nervous system day in and day out. This can only lead to elevated cortisol levels, which can lead to fatigue and burnout. Conversely, the parasympathetic nervous system allows us to rest and digest. It allows for a good 7-9 hours of deep uninterrupted sleep. It allows for a healthy appetite, enables us to digest food effectively, helps to keep our moods on an even keel and supports our microbiome. The important thing to recognize here is which nervous system you choose to engage most routinely is a choice.

Yes, a choice.

While sometimes we cannot choose the environments that we work in, live in, eat and breathe in, we do have the ability to decide how to manage it. Many have been programmed to believe otherwise, but we do choose to get stressed out or not. Stress is a two-way street; meaning when we are stressed, we also generally eat poorly. When we eat poorly it is stressful to our body. We have the ability to choose the foods that we put in our bodies, what we listen to, and the people we spend time with. We choose our reactions or responses to these environments. If a person or place that you routinely spend time with or around stresses you out, why would you continue to spend time with them or in that place? Many times, however, we have been doing things a certain way for so long that we become desensitized to stress because it's a habit. Only when our health fails do we start asking questions.

Stress will show itself in a variety of different ways in our bodies. Some folks will eat more, stop exercising, and gain weight. Others may experience gas, bloating, and diarrhea or get a stomachache and lose weight. Others may have a rise in blood pressure along with some of these other symptoms, and some may just develop neck pain and a headache from muscle tension or experience lack of sleep. Everyone's a little bit different. Most manifestations will impact nutritional status on some level. Ever notice you get sick more frequently when stressed? Stress can weaken the tight barrier in the intestinal tract that keeps harmful bacteria from entering your bloodstream. It can also allow larger parti-cles or less broken-down proteins to enter your system, potentially causing addi-tional disruptions, particularly to the immune system. Our bodies can usually handle a little stress but at the potential expense of low chronic inflammation. Remember my discussion about inflammation as a promoter of disease and autoimmune rates rising?

Without going into great detail, some of the nutrients that might be affected include B vitamins (higher need in diabetes or insulin resistance), magnesium (with some forms of IBS), vitamin C (required to produce a stress hormone called cortisol), and Vitamin D, omega 3 fatty acids, and tryptophan (necessary to produce serotonin, a neurotransmitter that helps with mood stabilization). These are just a few of the nutritional limitations that can occur from not manag-ing stress. Also, stress, by itself, can cause changes in the microbiome, which when left unattended can support chronic dysbiosis. If we couple this with a Standard American Diet (SAD) and its potential for malnutrition, we have a perfect storm for ill health.

Where should we turn to for help? Of course, the first place one should look is internally. What decisions can you make differently to influence your situation? If you need additional help, it's important to engage a practitioner in your area who knows and understands the nuances of improving health in your particular location. Depending upon the location in which you live, your stressors will be different. If living in a big city or next to a CAFO or the high-way, air quality could be impacting your health. If you live in a food desert on a limited budget, food access could be impacting your health. In certain parts of the country, water quality from public water supply or groundwater affected by local agricultural operations could be impacting your health. Mold in our houses can also be a contributor to poor health. Certain regions of the country are more prone to this. Beyond that, engage a practitioner who wants to find the root cause of your health concern rather than prescribing one more pill to ease a symptom. Remember, pain or discomfort is a *gift* that's telling you something's wrong. Don't ignore it.

Call the Right Kind of Doctor!

Finding a physician who can help manage medical care in a more holistic manner is essential for a long, healthy, active life. Don't be afraid to interview your physician. If it offends them that you would like to do this, you may need a different physician. If my clients want to become more aggressive with nutritional care, I recommend trying to work with the physician you have first, especially if your physician is one whom you have a good working rapport with. If interested in working on overall health from the nutrition or more holistic standpoint, the more an individual's care is worked in cooperation with your MD or DO the better. MDs or medical doctors focus more on allopathic medicine or medicine managed with medications. DOs or Doctors of Osteopathy may be more likely to work with you as a patient holistically because their training, while still conventional, is geared more toward prevention. This doesn't mean that your MD wouldn't be interested in looking at food as medicine, so having this discussion with them is still important. Conversely, it doesn't mean that just because you have a DO that they'll be willing to work with a dietitian or on holistic care. You see why the interview is so important.

There are also MDs and DOs who have obtained advanced certifications that focus on what's called Functional Medicine. Functional Medicine essentially looks at the body as a whole and tries to determine the root cause of illness rather than reducing the body into different unrelated systems that don't affect one another. It also embraces addressing the root cause of illness rather than just the symptoms. This is important in the effort to cure rather than just mask symptoms or as you'll hear me say frequently, "put a Band-Aid on the wound of someone who has had open heart surgery." Many doctors who have Functional Medicine certifications also understand the importance of food as medicine and will guide you toward farmers' markets as well as toward regenerative agriculture. Functional Medicine doctors are taught how to look for the root cause of illness from the system's biology standpoint and should be having discussions about how your life can be healthier holistically.

Some of these doctors may include genetic, stool testing, Cardio IQ testing (the types of cholesterol, LDL, HDL, not just a basic panel), inflammatory markers, food sensitivity testing, oxidative stress markers, hormone testing, waist-to-hip ratios, or the need for digestive enzymes as a part of their in-office assessments. This is important because one size doesn't fit all, and understanding your particular genetic circumstance can be useful for defining your own road map to health. Just as one size doesn't fit all nutritional care, neither does one size fit all medical care.

Additionally, don't limit yourself to just the conventional medical care providers. Other practitioners of evidence-based medicine are out there who can help guide you. Depending upon your circumstance, look for guidance also from Naturopathic, Chiropractic, Ayurvedic, Mediation, or Yoga practitioners. Just remember, if what you're doing isn't working, find someone who can help weed through the signs and symptoms of your medical concern to figure out the root cause of the problem.

I've worked with thousands of people who've become very frustrated with their medical care because they chose an allopathic physician and took their advice for a very long time. While you should be able to trust your physician, if you don't feel better after a visit to the doctor, have not developed a game plan for moving forward toward remediation/intervention for your health, the list of medications that have different side effects has become increasingly long, and are struggling to get the referrals you need, it may be time to consider an alternative approach. Remember that this is the steering wheel of your health. Make sure you point your vehicle in the right direction.

8.
Not All Who Wander Are Lost

When we embark on any new journey, perhaps the most daunting task is where to start. When it comes to our health, there's usually a directive. One that we have either imposed on ourselves or, if fortunate, with the aid of a professional who can help to guide us in the right direction. A good clinician, as discussed previously, will help establish goals and provide an actionable plan for how to get to the goals. For instance, if your goal is weight loss, after a thorough history and exam so the goals can be measurable, there would be interventions set in place to perhaps reduce calories, increase exercise, eat less junk food and address underlying nutritional deficiencies, if any.

This portion of our journey is less targeted than a therapeutic intervention with a healthcare clinician. Every human being on the planet has different thoughts, desires, concerns and attitudes, and this one-size-fits-all approach to healing our bodies just doesn't work. As a dietitian, my job is to tell people what to eat and perhaps which supplements to heal their bodies. This is what I have done for over 30 years. People go home, start a "diet" for a few days or perhaps a week and some even months before they call back and say they have fallen off the wagon and ask for help?" Sound familiar? What I want you to do here is to put your car in park for just a moment and reflect on why the diet didn't work. Insert a word or phrase into the blank here. My "diet" didn't work because_____. Was it a circumstance that influenced your diet? Divorce, challenging children, and toxic work relationships are some of the most common reasons that I hear in practice. Some mindlessly fall out of the plan put in place stating, "I'm not sure why I stopped doing it." Life happens. The actual reason it didn't work was because it wasn't the easy choice. The right choice or healthy choice has to be the easy choice or it won't continuously be chosen.

If you were to come to me to ask for help, one of the many things that we would discuss is that everyone is committed to something. If we're calling the food that we should normally be eating a "diet," we were never committed to the lifestyle changes that it takes in order to be successful with eating well over a lifetime. With your car still in park, ponder this. Why were we not committed to it? Was it not important enough? What were the obstacles to achieving what was set out as the goal? Everyone will have a different answer and, in any given circumstance, the answer may change. I'm going to suggest, however, that regardless of your answer, had you set in place the behaviors around eating well, your circumstance would become less significant. As human beings, we all deviate from the planned route on occasion, but if our eating behaviors are well established, then we get right back on with the journey and don't look back.

Now, put your car in reverse. We're going to back into how to functionally establish a lifestyle that keeps you eating well. This piece got lost a long time ago, perhaps decades, so this is why food becomes a free-for-all and fast food thrives today. The foundation of our health is bypassed because, as we previously discussed in Chapter 2, we're a society of convenience now. Our food environments don't support our health. Some people aren't in a place where they can purposefully change what they have to manage in a day; however, we can decide where and how we spend a portion of it. If we commit to spending it in ways that can potentially support health, then we change our health outcomes. We can change whether we eat well or not, which is one of the largest contributors to our health equation. These are the behaviors that we need to reestablish in order to commit to eating well, a lifestyle that maintains our health over the long term. But I want you to view it in this way. Below are 10 recommendations for engaging with your food in a foundational and fun way.

Of these 10 recommendations, the only recommendation that should be considered an absolute requirement for establishing new behaviors is the first recommendation. This is because all food behaviors stem from it. Otherwise, wander through the recommendations and decide what you can realistically take on in your circumstance. Not everyone follows the same road to good health. Talk with your family and friends who are also concerned about maintaining or improving their health. See how you can work together to create a new food environment for you, your family, and your friends who are interested in eating well, not just settling hunger pains but establishing Healthy Food Roots.

Healthy Food Root/Route #1 - **Define and Align Your Own Food Policy With Your Actions**

Huh? Sounds a bit formal. Let me explain further. Our personal food policy defines what we as individuals, are committed to with regard to food and food behaviors. Remember the discussion about commitment and our internal food narrative? The definition of policy is "a course or principle of action adopted or proposed by a government, party, business, or *individual*." Still sounds formal and a little scary. But here's the crux of it: our personal external and internal policies for our lives whether written down or psychologically acknowledged dictate our actions. In clinical practice and particularly when it comes to food behaviors, the stated belief system or even education level regarding food often don't match up. External is what we live out in our lives; that which we're acting on. Internal is what we've actually bought into on a personal level of which we sometimes aren't even aware. This internal commitment/policy or lack of commitment/policy doesn't necessarily exhibit itself externally. Essentially, words and actions need to match up in order to be successful.

For instance, I've worked with people who say they understand that eating vegetables is important for maintaining health. They like vegetables, but when I do a diet history, they eat one maybe two servings per day. Some folks even have wonderful and distracting stories about this one vegetable dish that they absolutely love that's made with super healthy ingredients. We know that eating more vegetables is important for good health, so where's the disconnect? Why are they only eating this fantastic dish only twice a year (assuming it's healthy of course)? Why does knowing that more vegetables are important for health not translate to eating more vegetables?

Before you read any further in this book, define your own food policy. Decide what's important to you as an individual or your family regarding what to put into or not put into your body. This is a very big deal. Now that you know more about the food in our food supply, what personal food policy can you realistically adopt in your circumstance that would be a step in a positive direction? Once defined, add actionable and measurable ways to ensure that you empower yourself to maintain your own policy. Think about what food behaviors or barriers you've had in the past to achieve moving forward with food decisions. No one can do this for you. This isn't to say that your policy motivation isn't influenced by other people, but your policy is your policy. This is yours and yours alone, which can either seem empowering or daunting, depending upon your mindset. Let's make this a little easier with a worksheet to work through with some food behavior ideas.

Define (Where am I headed?)

I want to make healthier food in my home.
I want to eat less fast food.
I want to eat less junk food.
I want to eat at least 5 servings of fruits and vegetables per day.
I want to eat more organic foods.
I want to eat more clean foods.
I want to eat fewer processed foods (no food label policy).
I want to support local farmers who farm with regenerative practices so I can be healthier and support the environment.
I want to learn how to cook on a lower budget.

What limitations do I currently have?

Financial limitations - food budget of $300 per month
I only have access to a car one day a week.

Time constraints - both my husband and I work full time on opposite shifts to save daycare expenses for our two children.

My husband isn't supportive of my desire to change my health.

It's just me in the house and I don't like to cook.

There's limited access in my area because I live in a food desert.

Align (How am I going to get there? Set realistic expectations.)

I'm going to shop at the farmers' market twice a month when in season.

I'm going to cook from scratch three evenings a week at home.

Before going to the grocery store, instead of shopping for my usual dishes, I'm going to look online for alternatives that can be cooked from scratch.

I'm going to reach out to three friends and see if they're interested in getting together to cook and eat one day a week (or twice a month or once a month).

I'm going to research the food products I'm eating (based on information learned in this book).

I'm going to start reading food labels and educate myself about what I'm eating currently.

I'm going to plan ahead two days in advance for my shopping experience.

I'm going to buy new kitchen gadgets(This is a favorite of mine!)

Schedule It

Put the farmers' market on your calendar.

Carve out time on Sunday (any day will work) afternoons to look for recipes, put together a list, and get the groceries you need to cook during the week.

Put your cooking experience on the calendar.

Monday evenings is product review time.

Volunteer at the local community garden, Sierra Club, or water quality nonprofit event.

Once you define your policy and align it with actionable steps, do your best to not look back. Many people ruminate (grass-fed cow humor) over what they would have done if things were different. Choose not to stumble backwards over something that's behind you with the realistic, actionable steps you put in front of yourself. Do this with a purpose! As you read through the remainder of this book, you'll need to revisit this section because you may want to add some additional actionable, fun steps offered in the pages that follow. This doesn't mean that there won't be challenges or that you won't get off track on occasion, but remember your policy and stick with the actionable steps that move you in the right direction. Don't be afraid to modify your policy in the event that something isn't working for you or if you feel that you've set yourself up for failure. Don't confuse this, however, with making excuses to not do what you can attain but lack motivation to complete. In this case, find someone close to you who will help keep you accountable. You can also do this with other health behaviors like exercise, meditation, etc. The point is to keep moving forward on your journey and actionably LIVE your food policy.

Healthy Food Root/Route #2- **Find Your Tribe - Create One If Needed**

There's an old African proverb that says, "If you want to go fast, go alone; if you want to go far, go together." When we "diet," many times, we take on a direction alone. Personal accountability is a fantastic attribute to have. But what happens when we falter? Think back to the last time you went on a "diet" and it didn't work. What happened? We all have a similar story. Life happens and then we quit the "diet." We all falter at some point or another due to life circumstances whether that's stress induced, family, or just plain tired and don't feel like it. This falter, while out of our control at times, is sometimes the beginning of the separation of our actions from our personal food policy. This is where the tribe comes in. They help to maintain engagement in a supported lifestyle.

Tribes:

1. Help to hold you accountable

2. Help out sometimes when you can't help yourself

3. Are truthful with you even when you don't want to hear it sometimes but not judgmental

4. Are inspiring, uplifting, and encouraging rather than demeaning and negative

5. Have routine contact

6. You can be honest with them about what you're struggling with; they're a safe place

7. Function with reciprocity

Reciprocity means the practice of exchanging things with others for mutual benefit. It's the give and take of life. Conceptually, it's also what builds strong communities. Our tribe can be family, friends, neighbors, coworkers, or people in places that we volunteer. Developing a tribe is a nonlinear process, meaning you don't just go fill out an application and find a tribe. It takes investment of time and energy as well as vulnerability to open ourselves up to one another and discuss what our actual needs are that we're struggling with.

Sometimes, it's helpful also to define something by explaining what it's NOT. Here are some examples of what a tribe doesn't look like that I've come across in clinical practice.

1. Visiting with a friend over tea when there's a give and take of the communication, but when they leave, you feel drained and anxiety ridden.

2. Your husband or wife says, "Honey, I'm 100% supportive of you and what you're trying to do with your new lifestyle!" But they then come home every evening from work and sit in front of the TV or computer screen, expecting to be fed or bring a bag of fast food.

3. Taking on all the care for an individual because you know you can handle it, which then doesn't allow you to take care of yourself.

4.   A friend who routinely says they'll help you to do the cooking but then doesn't ever follow through.

5.   A group of friends who love to get together but when they do, eat poorly, laugh, and justify it.

Trust is built through words and actions matching up. Building trust takes time and consistent action over time.

We know from research how important socialization is, especially following the COVID-19 pandemic. The natural progression of social distancing became, for some, social isolation, which led to stress eating and then weight gain and further distancing due to embarrassment for some. I suspect there will be a body of literature that will examine its impact on not just our physical but mental health as well.

Volunteering is a great way to help build a tribe and help our health also. In Canada, an Ontario study on volunteering linked to health benefits found that volunteering not only improves self-esteem but also helps to reduce social isolation, lower blood pressure, and enhance the immune system.[116] Furthermore, volunteering also reduces mortality in older adults. When people gather together over community causes and work together to accomplish goals, it has a tendency to bond people for life. Have you ever gone to a volunteer event and noticed how you felt when you left? Offering your time without expecting anything in return reaps great benefits for you as well as the organization to which your time is offered. And you just went there to have fun and help out!

---

[116] Thompson, R. Gardening for Health: A Regular Dose of Gardening. *Clinical Medicine*. 2018 Jun; *18*(3): 201-205. https://www.ncbi.nlm.nih.gov/pmc/articles/PMC6334070/

Healthy Food Root/Route #3 - **Identify Programs and Community Initiatives Within Your Area that Support Your Personal Food Policy**

Here is where we put some feet to our personal food policy. Please remember that we all need to be supported in order to be effective. No man or woman is an island. Write down what you want to accomplish this year with your health. The best way to teach this is by example. Let's say that our goals are to:

1. Increase vegetable consumption.

2. Become more aware of the foods we eat and their environmental impact.

3. Lose 10 pounds by the end of the year.

4. Plant some herbs and use those herbs in recipes at least once a week.

5. Work with your church and/or family to try to increase access to healthy food options.

If one of your health goals is to eat more fruits and vegetables or to become more environmentally conscious and you live in the city, search for urban agricultural programs in your location. Not only is working in the soil healthy for the microbiome but any form of urban agriculture builds community capacity by providing skills beyond growing food. There are now plenty of studies that support how urban agriculture can increase local food production but also improve food literacy skills, social relationships, physical activity, and pride in community settings.[117] [118] Community vegetable gardens can induce significant,

---

[117] Garcia, M. T., Ribeiro, S. M., Germani, A. C. C. G., & Bógus, C. M. The Impact of Urban Gardens on Adequate and Healthy Food: A Systematic Review. *Public Health Nutrition*. 2018 Feb; *21*(2): 416-425. https://www.ncbi.nlm.nih.gov/pubmed/29160186

[118] Martin, W., & Vold, L. Building Capacity Through Urban Agriculture: Report on the Askîy Project. *Health Promotion and Chronic Disease Prevention in Canada*. 2018

positive behavioral changes among its members, particularly associated with the environment.(118,119) Awareness of the environment's high social priority and increased consumption of organic food, fruits and vegetables usually, helps foster these relationships.(119) These people could essentially become a part of your tribe.

Community Supported Agriculture or CSAs are also a way to connect in this capacity. So not only can you support by voting with your fork (Healthy Food Root/Route #8) but some CSAs are set up for members to work on the farm for a deferred cost. Every CSA is different, so make sure you review the options for seasonality, overall cost, and what the CSA actually offers. Some offer just on-farm produce. Some offer baked goods and value-added products such as jams and jellies or salsa. Some provide weekly flowers in addition to the food, which is a nice touch. Engage with these programs, and your perception of growing food vs. what you see on the shelf of the grocery store and how it got there will also change.

Community gardens also offer a variety of opportunities to connect with food. Just like CSAs, they're all a little different so do your research in the area you live. See what opportunities exist and what level of involvement you can invest. Some simply offer opportunities to garden with a group in large gardens, others an opportunity to produce your own food in a plot that you rent, and yet other more developed programs offer classes on how to garden and even do cooking demonstrations with the food that they grow. Some accomplish this regeneratively, some not but regardless of how they're run, most community gardens will offer an opportunity to increase fruit and vegetable consumption as well as reduce food costs.[119]

Jan; *38*(1): 29-35. https://www.ncbi.nlm.nih.gov/pmc/articles/PMC5809110/

[119] Nova, P., Pinto, E., Chaves, B., & Silva, M. Urban Organic Community Gardening to Promote Environmental Sustainability Practices and Increase Fruit, Vegetables and Organic Food Consumption. *Gaceta Sanitaria*. 2020 Jan-Feb; *34*(1): 4-9. https://www.ncbi.nlm.nih.gov/pubmed/30471837

In Springfield, Missouri, we have a food bank called Ozarks Food Harvest (OFH). They service 200 food pantries in and around SW Missouri. While feeding hungry stomachs, food pantries are notorious for providing unhealthy, nonperishable food products that have a very long shelf life. What's special about OFH is that they have engaged in the local food scene and offer a program that provides assistance to local farmers called the Glean Team and also have their own gardens in an attempt to offer healthier food options to folks who have access to a kitchen to cook or process these foods, The Glean Team, when called, will go out to a local farm and help that farmer harvest a crop in a hurry. The most common gleaning requests were due to inclement weather that would completely ruin a crop due to hail or frost if not harvested. This helps both the farmer and OFH, which would then purchase the crop for a reduced rate and provide it through their distribution center. They also allow volunteering at their Full Circle gardens. Both of these opportunities provide experiences that help people connect more with food.

OFH helps to address food insecurity by providing over 15 million meals per year to people in need. They're an affiliate of Feeding America. While the trend is toward food banks having more perishable-based food programs, not all have the same opportunities as OFH. But don't be afraid to inquire in and around the area in which you live.

One of the most underutilized resources is Extension Services. Traditionally Extension has been in every county across the US but there are now only approximately 2900 offices. We're very fortunate in Missouri as funding has been maintained for every Extension office in our state, all managed through the University of Missouri. In other states, it will be managed through in-state higher learning facilities so all one needs to do is google Extension and the state or county that they live in to find resources immediately available to you. In many cases, these offerings are without a charge and therefore only cost some time and energy. Online courses, with titles including The Beginning Gardener, Getting Started with Vegetables, Healthy Yards for Clear Streams, as well as other publications like Beekeeping Tips for Beginners, Vegetable Planting Calendars, Improving Habits for Wildlife in Your Backyard, Adventures in Nutrition with the Show

Me Chef, Preserve it Fresh/Preserve it Safe (home canning), and many others are available.

Master Gardener programs are also administered through Extension in Missouri and also offer volunteer opportunities to maintain Master Gardener status. These classes cost some money but after 30 hours of class time, you'll have a good base of knowledge for how to grow your own food.

Future Farmers of America (FFA) is also managed through Extension. FFA is usually affiliated with local school systems and the strength and enthusiasm for the programs comes from the Ag Teachers within the public school system. It's usually an elective class so encouraging children toward being involved with these programs is essential because, many times, they're not even aware of these opportunities.

Additionally, pretty much anywhere in the USA has concerns about food insecurity on some level. Are you a member of a church that has the same concerns about access to food and are interested in starting your own community garden in cooperation with the church? Many churches recognize this as a community concern and want to do something to help. If one of your goals is to learn how to grow some food, then having the support of a congregation and information from Extension makes the task seem a little less daunting. If the garden takes off, it's also possible to obtain grant money from USDA via EQUIP loans that will essentially pay for a high tunnel, a large greenhouse, as long as there has been food grown in that location prior to the application being submitted. Many hands make light work.

In Springfield, we have a nonprofit that supports community outreach and education around food called Simple Organized Savings (SOS). SOS has classes on life skills, hydroponics for kids, couponing, strategic shopping, cooking and freezing, as well as time management. On their front page it encourages, "We were never designed to do life alone! Let us come alongside you so you can organize your family first, then go out and impact your community." Never were there more true words. Sometimes, it takes one person to plant that seed that then becomes a community, statewide, national, or global movement. If one of your goals is eating healthier on a lower budget, finding a resource such as this in your location is one more level of support to meet individual goals.

As previously mentioned, local food programs many times overlap to some degree with water quality initiatives within a region. The reason for this is that water quality within a region is affected by local agricultural endeavors and can have either a positive or negative impact.

In SW Missouri, we have some well-established 501c3 nonprofits dedicated to water quality. The Watershed Committee of the Ozarks (WCO) https://watershedcommittee.org/about-us/ and the James River Basin Partnership (JRBP) https://www.jamesriverbasin.com/ both have some consistent volunteer opportunities that help unite people with the source of their water quality. Make a plan with a friend to attend a volunteer opportunity or program to learn what you might be able to do personally. Water quality affects absolutely everyone. A friend of mine who used to be the President of JRBP once said, "Ange, food is important but water is more important. You can go 3 weeks without food but only 3 days without water and food doesn't grow without water." And if one really thinks about it, if we're, in fact, drinking the amount of water that we should, the quality of our water may have a greater impact on our health than food. Remember the discussion about water quality in Chapter 3? I personally am a stickler for high quality water for this reason, and that's why I support both these organizations. While this may not directly affect dietary food intake, it will certainly make you begin to think about what influence you can personally have, while on this planet. Some of their outings involve quite a bit of physical activity as well.

Another great way to support your health is to shop at local farmers' markets. In Chapter 4, I discussed how to choose local food. Here's your chance to execute! Many local farmers' markets are taking the approach that while the market supports mainly local food and food items, they're allowing other value-added products and services that give it more of a destination appeal. Come shop at the farmers' market, eat some fresh baked goods, have some coffee from a local roaster (some markets allow for local businesses to come in, even though there are no local coffee growers), hang out and listen to some music and visit with a friend. Spending a few hours at the market may mean a consumer/eater is more likely to have that conversation with the farmers about how they're growing and raising food on their farm. Farmers' markets also have events to pull people to their markets, making it a destination for the day. Make sure you google some of the markets that are close to you and see what events they have coming up.

One of our most successful markets in SW Missouri is the Webb City Farmers Market. The Webb City market has been successful because they found creative ways to support their vendors. They have a certified kitchen available for producers to create their own value-added products as well as classes to help support their growers. They also normally have a calendar of creative events providing opportunities for children and adults alike. How does this improve your health? It provides the opportunity to build a relationship with your farmer, socializing away from electronics and in a fun and food-centric environment. The moral of the story is: find additional ways to connect yourself with your food that keeps you moving forward with your goals!

Healthy Food Root/Route #4 -
Attempt Agritourism!

One of the most fantastic ways to build a relationship with food is to engage with the people who produce it. Agritourism is essentially where tourism and agriculture meet. Many states have their own websites for encouraging agritourism: https://www.visitmo.com/trip-ideas/agritourism-adventure. Additionally, many farms have on-site BNB operations, U-pick opportunities, tours, festivals, cheese or wine making, yoga among some of the more docile farm animals, educational or farm-to-table dinner events. In Missouri, there are plenty of opportunities to seek additional adventure that center around farm living. If you're planning to travel or just looking for a unique local experience, many of these opportunities are just around the corner from your house.

Where I live in SW Missouri, I purposefully try to reach out to local food business owners in an attempt to build a relationship with them. Some of the more enjoyable visits have been when producers are in their down season (usually winter) which is relative to the individual operation because they have more time to visit. One rainy Saturday, I ventured out to a local winery in Seymour, Mo called Lambs and Vines, http://www.lambsandvineswinery.com/mesmerize/our-story/. It drew my attention because of the story behind their attempt at organic wine production in Missouri. They allow their Babydoll Southdown sheep to graze in and among the grapevines as a way to support a symbiotic relationship between animals and the earth that the grape vines grow in. Their dream and story is encouraged with some success but also fraught with failures over the years, including one year when the sheep consumed all the profits! But they didn't give up! In their tasting room, they also have wool products for sale as well as some wine and cheese to nibble with your wine selection if one were to desire to stay and visit for a bit overlooking the grapes and the valley.

Another great example in SW Missouri is Millsap Farms. Curtis Millsap and his wife Sarah own a 20-acre farm on the north side of Springfield. They've been operating the farm since 2005. Once a month, they offer free Twilight Farm Walks that speak to the on-farm operations, vision, and connection with the earth. Mid-May through October, they also offer wood-fired pizza nights on Thursday evenings. The pizza toppings are mostly vegetable toppings from food that was grown on the farm or locally sourced. These are fun, music-filled evenings that exemplify how a community can come together, produce great food, and have a good time doing it. They also have a self-service farm stand and CSA where they sell not only their own food but also flowers, offer value-added products and other farmers' products as well. Millsap Farms also puts out a variety of videos about transparency with their food products. They raise food regeneratively and, as we've learned previously, this is important because this is clean eating. And the transparency allows us to choose what we want to put into our bodies.

The next time you take a trip and are planning where to stay, google Airbnb or VRBO and when the additional filters pop up, look for opportunities that involve BnB experiences or on farm/farmhouse experiences. Many times, these folks are providing meals with some of the products produced on the farm and would enjoy an opportunity to share their vision behind ensuring that they're providing not just food on a table but a food experience. There may be fewer overnight options, but I can almost guarantee that you'll enjoy the experience.

Healthy Food Root/Route #5 - **Grow Something….. Anything!**

For those of you who grow food in some capacity, I don't need to explain why this is a great idea. For those of you who think this seems a little silly or perhaps daunting, the reason you need to grow something is because, just like any investment, it connects you to your food. The reconnection with real food is what's needed in our society today. We love our trendy food products, but only real food supports our health. When a seed is planted in the soil, it's watered every few days, and eventually when it starts peeking up through the soil, the delight for anyone who partakes in this event is unmeasurable as far as connecting with our food. It's an investment in time, energy, and enthusiasm that feeds the soul. Minimal efforts can produce great and lasting results that provide a culinary offering that gives and gives.

There are now studies about how growing a garden can improve your health. Garden therapy is now becoming known as Green Care. Green Care has been used in other countries such as Norway and the Netherlands as intervention for folks with impaired mental health as well as drug dependence. In the UK, Green Care or Care Farming is offered on a large scale as a response to escalating concerns over health and social issues such as obesity, depression, prison overcrowding, recidivism, and a disaffected younger generation.[120] Care farming involves the use of commercial farms and agricultural landscapes as a base for promoting mental and physical health, through normal farming activity. It has flourished as partnerships between multiple sectors including health care, social services, public health, and educators provide structured care services

---

[120] Green Care or Care Farming website. https://www.farmgarden.org.uk/knowledge-base/article/what-care-farming

centered around the agricultural setting. The interesting part of this is that this started separate from any policy support from the government, meaning that the different sectors noted that there was a need and addressed it without financial support or subsidization.

Care farmers report that the physical benefits experienced by clients include improvements to physical health and farming skills. Mental health benefits consist of improved self-esteem, well-being, and mood, including an increase in self-confidence, enhanced trust in other people and calmness. Examples of social benefits reported by care farmers are independence, formation of a work habit, the development of social skills and personal responsibility.[121]

Why is gardening so healthy? It's most likely the combination of the physical activity, social interaction, and the exposure to sunlight as well as being in nature in general. Spending time outside reduces the amount of exposure to screen time, which, in turn, can help to reduce rates of depression.[122] Not only this but the availability of more healthy food now exists. When you grow your own food, you're more likely to eat it!

Real, garden-fresh food can be grown on a small scale in a container on a back or front porch as well as in a backyard garden. Some people have access to community garden plots for minimal cost or a larger backyard garden by the acre. No matter what you have available to you, there's a way to grow something. If there are foods or herbs that you routinely purchase at the grocery store, consider

[121] de Boer, B., Hamers, J. P., Zwakhalen, S. M., Tan, F. E., Beerens, H. C., & Verbeek, H. Green Care Farms as Innovative Nursing Homes, Promoting Activities and Social Interaction for People With Dementia. *Journal of the American Medical Directors Association.* 2017 Jan; *18*(1): 40-46. https://pubmed.ncbi.nlm.nih.gov/28012503/

[122] Khouja, J. N., Munafò, M. R., Tilling, K., Wiles, N. J., Joinson, C., Etchells, P. J., John, A., Hayes, F. M., Gage, S. H., & Cornish, R. P. Is Screen Time Associated With Anxiety or Depression in Young People? Results from a UK Birth Cohort. *BMC Public Health.* 2019 Jan 17; *19*(1): 82. https://www.ncbi.nlm.nih.gov/pubmed/30654771

growing them to supplement your grocery bill. A container garden can be started for less than $25 even if you're starting from scratch.

While this may seem like a lot of money for start-up, consider your weekly food costs, especially if choosing organic. Let's use rosemary as an example. A small one ounce cut of organic rosemary costs $3.99 at the grocery store. A full, small, plant from the store also costs $3.99. If not used quickly, the rosemary cuts will go bad in the fridge before using it again. If you plant a Rosemary plant in the ground, it will start growing and then it's available for your next recipe. You make up for your initial investment within two recipes if planted in the ground and if nurtured you may have that rosemary plant for years to come. If placed in a container, you recoup costs within five recipes and you have the convenience of having it on your back door step. The cost savings is tremendous for very little effort.

Herb and spice intakes can also improve health. Some studies suggest that only two TBSP per day can improve overall health.[123] They're concentrated forms, as they're mostly consumed dried, of antioxidants, anti-inflammatory, and glucose- and cholesterol-lowering medicinal food. A great way to "spice up" your life is to grow your own as you'll be more likely to find recipes to use it.

One year, I noticed that my purple sweet potatoes were sprouting eyes in the pantry. I figured I had nothing to lose but a few minutes of my time if I cut them up and put them in the ground. The vines were quite pretty as they started to grow out as were the lightly purple flowers toward the end of the season but oh the bounty that they provided my family and friends that year! Those few purple sweet potatoes turned into two 5-gallon buckets of sweet potatoes. This can also be done with any other kind of potato, garlic, and other foods at the right time of year. How fun it is to experiment with nature!

---

[123] Jiang, T. A. Health Benefits of Culinary Herbs and Spices. *Journal of AOAC International.* 2019 Mar 1; *102*(2): 395-411. https://pubmed.ncbi.nlm.nih. gov/30651162/

If growing from scratch, try heirloom quality plants and seeds. The reason for this is twofold. First, you support the folks that are trying to ensure that old-world seeds continue to be available. So, just like we vote with our food dollars, we vote with our seed dollars too. In Southwest Missouri, we have the great benefit of having several heirloom seed companies with one of the largest in the country, Baker Creek Seed Company, right here in Mansfield. Every year, they hold what's called the Spring Planting Festival the first weekend in May when thousands of people come from all over the country to listen to workshops on growing food, health, regenerative agriculture, seed gathering adventures, and folk music. There are also artisan vendors who provide garden-related products, seedlings, food products, and crafts. Every year, we brought our mobile pizzeria there to make pizzas for hundreds of people in this fantastically upbeat family-friendly atmosphere with people who share a common goal: growing their own food.

The second reason is that they reseed themselves. This is unlike genetically modified or hybridized seeds. Every year, I walk out into the garden and I have these nice surprises called volunteers. Volunteers are when a seed that's not purposefully planted in the garden starts to sprout. This usually comes from a fruit that wasn't picked up from the ground last year or it survived the decomposition from the compost pile from the previous year. If recognized as a food plant coming up in your garden rather than a weed, which happens the more you grow food, you can transplant it to a place that you want it to grow and enjoy the additional bounty that has been provided to you with little to no effort.

If growing something from seed seems intimidating to you, find a farm that offers plants, a planting festival, or a farmers' market near you, which usually have vendors selling seedlings or sprouted seeds. Larger box stores like Lowe's or Home Depot also have seedlings available, especially in the spring season. They may or may not be heirloom quality, but just getting started growing is the important message here.

If small container growing can supplement food dollars, think about what a larger garden can do. Be cautious with becoming overzealous, however, thinking that a 20-by-20-foot plot is a great first step. It's possible to try to attempt too much too quickly, so start small, plan and then expand. Bill Alexander's book, *The $64 Tomato: How One Man Nearly Lost His Sanity, Spent a Fortune, and Endured an Existential Crisis in the Quest for the Perfect Garden,* is a great example of what not to do with your first garden attempt. Start small, start composting from table scraps and involve your children, friends, or parents in what you're doing. It really doesn't matter what your age or income is, as everyone benefits from being involved, as long as it's not treated as one more thing to manage in our checklist of life.

If you already have a garden and want to start growing through four seasons, consider applying for an EQIP loan through the USDA. These loans are essentially for anyone that has an established garden who wants to take their home growing to a whole new level. Greenhouse growing requires an additional skill set so do your research and check out the loan options here, https://www.nrcs. usda.gov/wps/portal/nrcs/main/national/programs/financial/eqip/. It's offered through the NRCS or Natural Resource Conservation Service arm of the USDA. This past year, the loans didn't even have to be repaid.

Healthy Food Root/Route #6 - **Play with your Food!**

This is perhaps one of my most favorite Food Roots. The reason is because once a person learns how to have fun with their food, then their whole connection with food changes. It moves from one more thing that needs to be taken care of to a wonderful creative process that we make time for several times a week. I remember when I was kid and afraid to make a mistake in the kitchen mainly for fear of wasting food. This fed into the idea that it was easier and, as we've discussed, more convenient, to have someone else grow, gather, process, and make our food.

As I grew older, my disposition around food changed, however. It changed because I began to understand that the only way I was going to be "in charge" of my food was to make it myself from ingredients that I trusted. And the only way to ensure that I would be able and willing to sustain it would be to make sure it was fun! So here it is: PLAY WITH YOUR FOOD! No food fights please but if you're the primary housekeeper, that also will be your prerogative!

To be clear, this doesn't mean that every food you attempt to make is going to be a rockstar when the family gets together. But don't be afraid to try new recipes with different seasonal ingredients. You'll find that the more that you play with your food, the more you'll want to do it, as well as be able to put different, desirable flavors together without a recipe. Crossovers in the taste categories are the new way to tantalize the palate. Combinations of sweet/salty or savory, (think pineapple on pizza or rosemary infused honey) in the past several years has given way to culinary experiences that tantalize more of your taste buds to be activated so that your mouth bursts with flavor.

Scientifically, there are basically four taste categories: salty, sour, sweet and bitter. Recently there has been a fifth added called umami which explains a savory sort of flavoring naturally found in some foods. Chemically, however, it's specifically associated with a free form of glutamate that can occur naturally with fermentation, aging, curing, or even normal ripening of foods. In 1990, it was finally recognized as the fifth taste and then in 2006, University of Miami scientists located the actual taste bud receptors, which solidified its place as a taste. Most of us are familiar with the favorite flavor enhancer known as MSG or Monosodium Glutamate (remember Chinese Restaurant Syndrome?) which for some people can have some negative side effects if taken in large doses but otherwise remember that glutamate occurs naturally in food and otherwise doesn't necessarily cause the same side effects.

Here are some ideas for getting started:

1. Talk with some friends and decide on one night a week to get the kids together to play in the yard while the adults cook some food together. Try to maintain this over time.

2. Start your own food club if there are none in your location. This doesn't have to be formal. In fact, some of the more fun clubs are informal ones where folks compete with new food recipes.

Everyone votes for the winner at the end of the potluck and the winner gets a small prize.

3. Become your own informal gourmet. This used to scare me! What, no plan? Some great recipes come from throwing together food that you have in the fridge that you have no plan for when you're willing to experiment. Recently, I had a client of mine call it Guessipe Night. How fun!

4. Get together with a friend and cook a meal together. One person creates the entree and the other the sides. I split it this way just from the food cost standpoint, but there are no rules.

5. About groups getting together. Decide on a theme: Mexican, Thai, Italian, Greek, etc. Everyone brings a dish and a copy of their recipe. This provides an opportunity for a healthy sort of sharing and some competitiveness.

6. Choose easy recipes to play with to start. The less complicated with fewer ingredients the better when you're getting started. Make sure you have an accomplice, even if it's a child.

7. Learn how to make your own bone broth. It's super expensive to buy bone broth made from regeneratively raised animals. If you're buying regeneratively raised meats, making your own broth is a natural extension of this, which can be done with very little time and effort and then you can reap the benefits of having it on hand to make gut-healing soups and bases for other kitchen creations.

Share failures as well as successes. Everyone loves a good laugh about a messy kitchen, sauce splattered everywhere, the kombucha experiment that exploded because it was shaken before opening (I don't recommend doing this!) or the burnt entree that forced the whole family to go out to eat for the evening. No harm done. Becoming more secure in our food journey is perhaps the one thing that allows us to be most creative moving toward healthy eating options. In the book, *Neur-ish-ment*, I played with many recipes to provide examples of healthy food options that taste great. I was making a batch of the Spicy Purple Kraut in the book which I always looked forward to, but this particular batch was off. Disgustingly off, actually. I had read that if it smells funny you shouldn't eat it, which is a hilarious statement because all kraut smells funny. It's called sauerkraut for a reason, right? Until you experience bad kraut, only then can you relate. I learned what the experts meant that day and promptly relegated that batch to the compost pile.

Try to create or attend food experiences that everyone wants to show up for rather than simply providing meals for the family. Turn on some music while you cook. Invite some friends over to cook together. I have a friend who offers "Bourbon Dinners." Andreas Adkins of *Gourmet Goodness* puts together a five-course meal that's paired with different bourbons from around the world as well as a locally sourcing part of the meal. During one of these events, the beef farmer even came and talked about his product. They talked about the foods being served and the trials with production, so you connect with the delectable morsel on your plate rather than just eating calories or a piece of meat. These meals are an expensive version of what we all could achieve by looking at food as an adventure rather than a chore.

When I was a kid, I always looked forward to fondue night. This was one of those occasions when my father would cook, and everyone knew how much Dad loved to make classic Swiss fondue. It was always a challenge to be patient while smelling the crusty bread roasting slightly in the oven coupled with garlic that's initially smeared in the bottom of the pot before the wine and cheese were all melted together and simmered for the better part of an hour. As I aged, I began to offer help so I could learn all of his "how to" tricks as well as keep myself busy while my stomach was growling. Somehow, being in the middle of the production always makes the time pass more quickly. When we finally sat down for dinner everyone got to choose their color fondue stick so that there would be no confusion about which stick was whose when left to simmer in the pot at the center of the table. Inevitably, someone would lose their bread or vegetable in the fondue only to become a distant memory of what would have been another tasty morsel. To this day, 45 years later, we often have fondue night when the family gathers. These traditions are the foundations of our food fun.

Healthy Food Root/Route #7 - **Change One Food Behavior a Month**

When we take the 10,000-foot view of our lives, we can begin to identify some of the behaviors that affect our health. It's never easy to stand back and look at the behaviors that keep us unhealthy, but as Albert Einstein once said, "The definition of insanity is doing the same thing over and over and expecting a different result." This chapter is where we begin to identify some behaviors that may need to change in an effort to influence our overall health outcomes.

Where do we start? Keep it grateful. Studies show that gratitude, in particular, is important in maintaining our perspectives. Regardless of where we are in life, gratitude affects our physical and emotional health. Try writing down three things you're grateful for every evening. What you're grateful for doesn't have to have anything to do with food. Why is this considered a food behavior? Because this will help set the tone for the rest of your choices. Gratitude impacts our decision making with regard to relationships, enhances empathy, reduces aggression, aids in restful sleep patterns, and improves self-esteem and mental strength. It also impacts our wisdom around appreciating life experiences as learning opportunities regardless of how positive or negative. Sounds like a great place to start when trying to change food behaviors. I might also suggest that much of the reason why we don't change our food behaviors really doesn't have anything to do with the food itself. It's more the general behaviors and approach to life that impact our decision making around food. Most of us know what we need to do, but for some reason, cannot make ourselves do it.

Because food should be engaging, here are some additional ideas to keep it fun:

1. **Buy a new food gadget**! Start small like a new, very sharp knife. You can get a great sharp knife for $50. Buy a sharpener too! What that purchase will do for you if you keep that knife sharp is allow you the opportunity to look forward to cutting up vegetables! There's nothing more frustrating than pulling out a knife to cut a tomato and having

the knife bounce off the tomato or squish it because it's not sharp enough to cut it. Conversely, if it's sharp, the culinary experience can be quite enjoyable. The more you cook, the more you'll begin to identify other kitchen gadgets or utensils that you would like to have. Your experience and desires for creating new foods will dictate your next purchase. In my kitchen, some other essential equipment includes a coffee grinder, French press, whole peppercorn grinder, salad spinner, Vitamix, and a high-quality food processor. These last two make almost any recipe easy to accomplish. Some of my recipes I used to chop ingredients by hand now cut my food prep time in approximately one third by using these items. As busy as we are these days, this is incredible time savings!

2. **Substitute some store-bought items for homemade.** As we discussed in Chapter 4, many of the food additives in food have the ability to make us sick by disrupting our microbiomes, especially if we eat a lot of them. If you buy a lot of convenience food items, it may be time to try to make it from scratch. You might find that many of these items are quite easy to make from scratch and quite enjoyable if you have the right equipment. Good examples are items like hummus and guacamole. A good food processor is helpful to make the hummus, but the guacamole only requires a knife and a spoon if the avocados are ripe. Part of the food journey here is to learn how to choose a ripe avocado if you've never done this before. Here is a link to describe how to choose ripe avocados: https://loveonetoday.com/how-to/pick-buy-fresh-avocados/.

3. **Choose a food approach.** A one-size-fits-all approach to meal planning and the diet that we choose doesn't exist. Commit to whatever approach you decide. Are you going to try Keto? Please don't do this unless you're working with a physician). Or maybe you're going to eat Paleo, start eating breakfast at home, do intermittent fasting, or try Mediterranean-style eating. Whatever it is, start working through the logistics of your success. Mentally start walking through

your day tomorrow with regard to your new commitment. If you were to simply start eating breakfast, for instance, ask yourself if you have breakfast foods at home. Do you have the right breakfast foods at home? Do you need to get up earlier? How much earlier? Walk through how you plan to successfully manifest your food approach and go for it! If you make a mistake, don't let it bother you; call it a learning opportunity and move past it toward your health.

4. **Try a new vegetable every week.** Notice that this doesn't say, try a new meat product every week. Our Standard American Diet (SAD) is very low in vegetables. A new recipe coupled with a new vegetable would be a Win/Win. Some examples of less common vegetables would be jicama (great cut up and dipped in hummus), Swiss chard, fennel, kohlrabi, purple sweet potato, bitter melon, Romanesco, purple green beans (they turn green when cooked) and celeriac. These vegetables may even be found at your local farmers' market. Commit to mixing it up! Google a simple recipe and enjoy.

5. **Research a water filtration system.** Water is just as important to life as food. In fact, per unit of our human body weight, it should be the one thing that we consume the most. What water filtration system will work for your budget? I recommend reverse osmosis systems but not everyone can afford one. One of the places I start gathering information is the Environmental Work Group or EWG, https://www.ewg.org/tapwater/water-filter-guide.php. Start to research options. The EWG or environmental work group is a nonprofit that does product review and can help provide some guidance on where to start for your budget. Also, don't be afraid to call local water filtration system providers. Their job is to educate you on your potential purchase. Ask tons of questions!

6. **Start fermenting foods.** This is one of my most favorite new kitchen skills. It can also be one of the scariest because of what it is. We have been raised in a sterile society that believes on some level that bugs are bad, so to purposefully cultivate the bugs that are in the air that

we breathe as well as the food that we eat seems a bit out there. These bugs as previously discussed have a symbiosis with their environment and therefore are a part of the overall balance in our lives that essentially goes unrecognized. I remember the first time I brewed Kombucha. It started bubbling, hissing and wheezing. It was wheezing that made me think of the old sitcom, The Jeffersons. I named my kombucha SCOBY, Louise. Mr. Jefferson would always yell to his wife, "Wheezie!....." From that point forward, whenever I shared any SCOBY with a friend, I told the friend that they would have to name the SCOBY. Louise had many offspring, including Mike, Frank, and Retha. There are endless possibilities for fermentation. Carrot sticks, pineapple, kraut, mead, bread, kefir, Kimchi, kvass, and kombuchas. I started with kombucha because it was the least labor intensive and the one food item that I was drinking a lot of from the grocery store. When I started making my own, the cost saving was in the tune of $1,000 per year and the health benefits unquantifiable.

7. **Learn about the transparency behind different foods.** In Chapter 4, The Blind Leading the Blind, we discussed food transparency in America and found out that there's a lot that we don't know about our food. If you have a favorite food that was on the top 10 adulterated food list, start researching how to continue to eat that food and get the most bang for your buck so to speak. The top 10 list included olive oil, milk, honey, saffron, coffee, maple syrup, orange juice, apple juice, vanilla, and grape wines. This list is obviously not all encompassing. Start researching your food and try to find out more about how to obtain the purest form of what you're wanting to continue to eat. Be cautious, however, because some of the information that you may uncover will be staggering, and remember to just do the best you can with what you know. I like to drink red wine with some of my more elaborate meals because it really does enhance the flavor of foods and vice versa. When looking at wine labels it's difficult to be educated on every wine producer and the time and effort involved in trying to figure out whether or not to spend the money or not. I

found it exhausting. So, I use a company that does the legwork for you by only offering organic, regenerative or sustainably produced wines with no added sugar, pesticide free, and delivered to your front door! Problem solved!

So, stepping out of our perpetual cycles of doing the same thing and our health not improving is an important motivator for other steps forward. Start small and pick something that you know you can succeed with. Pat yourself on the back, rest in your accomplishment, and next month, pick another that seems achievable or fine tune the one you started further. From these examples, identify other opportunities to change additional behaviors that we might not have considered. Have fun with this and involve other people. It's also a great way to build your tribe.

Healthy Food Root/Route #8 - **Vote With Your Fork!**

As consumers in America, we rarely head to the grocery store planning to vote. But this is exactly what we're doing when we purchase **anything,** whether it's food, drink, clothing, or gasoline. We all watched gas prices plummet during the COVID crisis. The cost of crude oil per barrel actually went into negative numbers at one point because there was very little demand for it. Most of the world wasn't driving anywhere, except for essential personnel and services. Therefore, there was no demand, and the prices fell.

So, here's how this works. We live in America, which is built on capitalism. Capitalism according to Oxford is an economic and political system in which a country's trade and industry are controlled by private owners for profit, rather than by the state or country. What you purchase is a vote to keep that product on the market. Your vote tells the person who created the product that you like it. There are over 15,000 new products on the market every year. There's an over 90% failure rate on processed food products. There's a big, long arduous process involved in getting a product to market that takes approximately two years, but here's what I would like you to consider. Your vote to purchase that product is the single most important decision you could make as a consumer. And, based on some of what you've been learning here, read the food label and mindfully decide whether this is something you wanted to put into your body.

Here's something else to consider. Do you have to test market an organic sweet potato or a banana? No. There are certainly better and worse places to try to sell them. You don't see a whole lot of vegetables hanging out on convenience store shelves for a reason. Remember my discussion about community food environments? We have to create our own food environments. This aside, there's a whole different subset of skills associated with buying ripe produce at the grocery store if it's available. I advocate for buying high-quality seasonal produce from our local stores, farmers' markets, or neighbors and, once we've taken the time to ask the right questions and scrutinize ingredients, some minimally processed food products as well.

In order to purchase some easy food substitutions, you may have to spend some time at the local health food store. Most regions have at least one. Here, one can usually find some easy substitutions that can't be found at regular grocery stores. Some easy substitutions for regular food products to start with include grass-fed butter; grass-fed beef, lamb, or bison; pastured pork or free-range chickens and eggs; any organic produce; and other organic foods. The little stickers on organic produce should start with the number 9 and have five digits to be labeled as organic. If it starts with a number 8 with 5 digits, it has been genetically altered, and if it only has four digits it's conventionally grown. Regardless of where you're shopping, always remember to check the label, if there is one, and do the best you can with the information you have available to you.

Another way that we can decide where to spend our food dollars is to search out local food cooperatives and/or aggregations centers or Food Hubs that are purposefully supporting local, organic sustainable or regenerative produce and buy from them. https://www.ams.usda.gov/local-food-directories/foodhubs Here is the national directory for foods Food Hubs.

Community Supported Agriculture or CSAs are also another way to support local people producing local food. CSAs were previously mentioned in Food Root #3 as a means to support your own food policy, but it's also a way to vote with your fork. Check out https://www.localharvest.org/ for additional options in your area. So not only can you support by voting with your fork but some CSAs are set up for members to work on the farm for a deferred cost. Every CSA is different, so make sure you review the options for seasonality, overall cost and what the CSA actually offers. Some offer just on-farm produce. Some offer baked goods and value-added products such as jams and jellies or salsa. Some provide weekly flowers in addition to the food, which is a nice touch. Engage with these programs, and your perception of growing food vs. what you see on the shelf of the grocery store and how it got there will also change.

Healthy Food Root/Route #9 - **Be Part of the SOILution!**

The Soilution or soil solution is quite important in the health of our daily lives. Think about the summertime and the number of times a person touches the ground during a week. As an example, one year I was walking at the lake around a marina with my dog and my ankles started to swell and itch as did my dog's face. I asked at the marina, and they indicated that nothing had been sprayed but I was obviously having a histamine response to something that my ankles kicked up in the dirt as did my dog. It happened again the following week. Whatever it was has long since been washed into the lake no doubt. The daily decisions that we all make with regard to how we manage the earth make a big difference. Everyone plays a part.

When was the last time you walked around your yard or property looking for the context of good biology? Notice where your plants are growing well versus where they're not growing well. Notice where there may be compaction in your yard and nothing is growing. On your property, where does the water puddle when it rains? How long does it take to drain off? These areas in your yard have potential to go anaerobic or grow high amounts of the wrong bacteria and protozoa if left underwater. Also, notice where weeds or something is growing that you don't want to grow there. These are all potential examples of unhealthy biology in the soil. Growing healthy plants can only be supported by the right kind of organic matter and biology in your soil! Here are some good places to start connecting with your food and understanding how important the soil microbiome is to your health and the health of the plants around you.

1) *Replace biology in your yard or on your grass and in your garden rather than using chemicals, "icides," or inorganic fertilizers*

Many folks rely on chemicals, pesticides (or other icides), and inorganic fertilizers to keep their lawns and gardens green and weed free. A little-known fact is that, if the biology is replaced properly, then the weeds don't want to grow. So, replacing biology not only reduces time getting your knees dirty but also creates a setup for additional water retention, therefore, less watering for a higher-quality more resilient food product or lawn. It's also less expensive to do it this way over time. Replacing biology supports itself, meaning that as long as the biology is fed and isn't altered by some mechanical or chemical means, it will support itself over time. It limits the need for perpetual agricultural inputs or fertilizers. If in SW Missouri, look at what www.soil123.com has to offer or, nationally, consider outreaching to www.soilfoodweb.com. They'll help guide you in the proper ways to manage these sorts of regenerative solutions. Please don't buy compost teas or extracts that have been sitting on a shelf in a plastic container for who knows how long. Most likely, whatever is in there has gone anaerobic and may or may not be the biology that you necessarily want to replace.

2) *Buy organic or regenerative foods and start composting your food and yard waste*

This is way less complicated than one might think. Depending on the type of composting you choose it can also be a lot of fun and a learning opportunity for the whole family. Many families do this because they don't want to contribute to the landfill and save a little money on bringing compost in from somewhere else. This way, one can take charge of that process and become more food sovereign. In gardening circles, I've heard story after story about "bad compost" and failed gardens because of this. Compost has gotten a bad rap because of compost brought in that doesn't have the right mix of inputs to support the proper biology in the soil. Great compost, on the other hand, has the proper biology in it to support the growth of plants not weeds. Do some research and get started using the natural resources that you already have at your fingertips. Again, there really is no downside to this. Just a little extra effort and don't forget to reach out to the experts if you have questions.

3) *If you don't want to compost in your own yard, consider giving your food or yard waste to someone who does.*

In Springfield, we have an organization called the Springfield Compost Collective. For a small fee per month, they'll give you a container and come retrieve your compostables every week. To learn more about this visit https://www.springfieldcompostcollective.org/ This means that you can compost and still feel good that you aren't contributing to the landfill as well. Another Win/Win sort of situation. Google composting options in your area. Other cities across the country also do this.

4) *When gardening on a large or small scale, consider no till practices and leave no bare soil.*

This has become the new go-to on the gardening/growing front. The act of tilling actually disrupts the biology in the soil by 50%. While tilling is perhaps more aggressive, the act of pulling up a plant by the roots essentially does the same thing. To be honest, until the biology in the soil is improved this doesn't work because the annual plant roots that are left in the ground don't break down over the winter. Because of this, a lot of people give up because it appears that it doesn't work. No or poor biology means the composting process doesn't occur as rapidly. The more it's practiced the greater the biology, again, as long as there are no mechanical or chemical disruptions in the soil. Let Mother Nature work her magic!

The same goes for ensuring that there is no bare soil in your garden. It used to be thought that ground cover or other understory plants utilized too many of the nutrients in the soil and therefore the plants you want to grow do not grow as well. This is not true. The understory plants keep the soil from being exposed to the elements which in turn protects the soil by keeping the biology intact.

Remember the conversation about how to keep nitrogen, carbon and phosphorous in place rather than going somewhere else? This is a part of that process.

5) *When starting to build or begin yard projects, consider replacing the biology even if none of the above has been attempted.*

I was visiting a friend who was complaining about the fact that Bermuda grass was always growing in her bushes in the front yard. Not only that but the bushes weren't doing that well. These two things together are symptomatic of one cause but the only way to know for sure would be to do a soil test for the biology in the soil. When tested, it was found that proportionately there wasn't enough fungi relative to bacteria in her soil. The right types of fungi would help to balance out the bacteria in her soil, keep the Bermuda grass from wanting to grow under her shrubs as much as it's an early successional plant that loves a higher proportion of bacteria to fungi while the bushes prefer significantly more fungi. The addition of proper organic matter and fungi to the soil supported the growth of the bushes while keeping the Bermuda grass from wanting to grow back. And when it did, it pulled out quite easily.

Please remember, nonregenerative agricultural methods on a larger scale may create a much greater burden on our local water supply than the average backyard gardener but every little bit counts. And there really isn't a downside to looking at doing this. Higher vegetable garden yields along with less weeding and more resilient disease-free plants are a Win/Win/Win. Just like the dream of having children everywhere understanding that their body is their temple, if they understood what biology is good in the soil for growing what, we would have a whole new world ahead of us because these folks would be making the policy decisions over the next 10-20 years.

Regardless, any decrease in concentrations of "nutrients" running off of impervious surfaces draining into aquatic ecosystems, which increases sediment loads in and nearby local water sources, is beneficial to all. This increase in sediment loads from runoff makes treatment of drinking water more difficult while also affecting fish and other aquatic life in any given watershed. To be clear, the disproportionate or out-of-balance offering of nutrients, bacteria, and sediment causes a challenge to the ecosystem, as they're always there on some level. Missouri in particular has a lot of grazing land with farmers who allow their cattle to wade in the rivers. While it's kind of novel to be floating on the river with cows in the water, once aware of the potential environmental impact, it certainly lessens the nostalgia.

Healthy Food Root/Route #10 - **Think Global, Act Local**

While it's not really known who coined the phrase "Think Global, Act Local," it has been utilized by many great philosophers, mathematicians, urban planners, business owners, and environmental activists over the last 100 years. The understanding that humanity must have a broad, global perspective about what's influencing our lives but understand that each individual must embrace the portion of responsibility that is, in fact, in our control. As mentioned before, not everyone has a national platform to further change, but we can certainly influence our immediate environments on some level. Think Global, Act Local encourages "placemaking," which encourages people in their own communities to work collectively, paying attention to an area's unique physical, social, and cultural identity to support change. Here, it will be homed-in on agricultural and food endeavors that help to support the health of its citizens.

One of the simplest ways to execute this if you don't want to grow your own food is to support restaurants that source local, regeneratively or organically grown foods. In Springfield, we have several well-established restaurants that do this. Here, I would like to highlight two of the stalwarts in our city, Gilardi's Ristorante and Farmers GastroPub. James Martin owner of Gilardi's, chef, and head dishwasher, has on the front page of his website this statement:

> "We are growing food on every square inch of this property and, in 24 months we will be a national model for sustainable restaurants. This is not just a restaurant. The lasting legacy of this business will be that we make the Ozarks a better place to live, one date, one plate at a time."

If you ever get a chance to sit down and talk with James about his vision for the property and his restaurant, you'll quickly realize that he wholeheartedly believes in what he's doing with Gilardi's. He's even happy to talk about the products that he sources locally that aren't grown on the property. Specifically, the meat and animal products he tries to source from local farmers because raising beef on a third of an acre in the center of Springfield is just not feasible.

Gilardi's is rivaled closely by the Farmers Gastropub, whose owner Andy Hampshire is from England and carries the tradition of the classic English Gastropub, meaning essentially a pub that serves very high-quality food. The quality of food when you speak to Andy has to do with how close to home it's raised. The list of farms whereby he sources most of his food from can be found on the back of the menu. Some believe that the best burger in Springfield can be found here at the Farmers Gastropub. The portions aren't overwhelming and they're 100% grass-fed.

There's a movement afoot for restaurants such as these to also be placed within community developments called Agriburbia or Agrihoods. These "food-centric" communities are based on sustainable or organic agricultural farming developments with strong social engagement opportunities, agricultural education, and implementation of economic development strategies that support the healthy, active lifestyles of its members. Sounds a little bit like that island called Vitality from Chapter 2. The Urban Land Institute (ULI) in their 2018 publication entitled *Agrihoods: Cultivating Best Practices,*[124] discusses some of the benefits and challenges with these developments. For most of us as consumers, the added benefit of considering Agrihoods is that the housing is usually lower cost, there are social opportunities/hubs with like-minded people, and there is increased access to healthy food options. In the US, ULI identified Agrihoods in 27 states. Imagine everyone in a community could walk out their door and pick fresh salad greens and some extra herbs for some accent flavor for their supper

---

[124] Matthew, N. *Agrihoods: Cultivating Best Practices,* The Urban Land Institute (ULI), March 2019. https://americas.uli.org/wp-content/uploads/sites/2/ULI-Documents/Agrihoods-Final.pdf,

that evening or, at least, have access to it locally, perhaps even within walking distance. These sorts of community developments, Agrihoods, are the food environment that we talked about influencing our health earlier in the book.

Additional opportunities that some Agrihoods provide are educational programs for children via farm tours or outdoor classrooms. When working in pediatrics, I was consistently saddened by how little our children knew about food. This is a natural result of our current society whereby we only obtain food from the grocery store and is then served to us without any engagement around how it got there, where it came from, and why that food was served. Farm-to-school programs are helping to close that gap. Farm-to-school programs successfully increase access to local food, provide nutrition education, strengthen the economy around family farms, and help to cultivate community bonds. Check to see if your child's school has a farm-to-school program. Most funding for farm-to-school programs actually comes from private and foundation donors, so consider a possible donation here as part of a local act of support.

Another fantastic way to engage children with their food is to help initiate a school garden. In Springfield, pioneering efforts were spearheaded by a now defunct organization called SUAC (Springfield Urban Agriculture Coalition). SUAC obtained funding for the The Dig in R-Twelve or DIRT project, working in cooperation with the Springfield school system to put 11 gardens in area schools. Because it would be a lot of work for one teacher to maintain within a location, DIRT helped create core garden teams to help maintain the gardens as well as develop teaching curriculum around the gardens. These sorts of programs are essential for teaching children about a relationship with food. Ideally, as with the DIRT project, sustainable or regenerative organic agriculture practices would be used. While following this particular program, the fantastic stories of children going home and teaching their parents about where their food came from and how to grow it, fostering additional healthy attitudes toward food, were immeasurable. These are great programs that help to combat the number one health problem for children in America: obesity.

In 2013, as an organizing effort to help combat childhood obesity in our region, I helped to spearhead the startup of the Ozarks Regional Food Policy Council or ORFPC. The ORFPC was formed in cooperation with the YMCA in Springfield as well as the hospital system CoxHealth. The belief was that our food systems were influencing healthy food availability in our region. As a part of our initiating efforts, we accomplished the first food assessment done within the region that identified the strengths, weaknesses, opportunities, and threats to a healthy food system. From this assessment, we were then able to make recommendations for next steps for our community about where to support our food system. Many organizations, for-profit and nonprofit, were then able to take those recommendations and walk forward to obtain further funding because there was now a plan put in writing.

Food Policy Councils (FPCs) are important because they support policy, which can provide positive support for local food initiatives. FoodFirst: Institute for Food and Development Policy makes the statement on their website, "The central aim of most Food Policy Councils is to identify and propose innovative solutions to improve local or state food systems, spurring local economic development and making food systems more environmentally sustainable and socially just." Food policy councils can be grassroots like the ORFPC or part of a government mandate. Some food policy councils engage heavily in politics, but the essential components of effective FPCs are strong leadership, strong community ties, and good organizational skills. There are food policy councils all over the country. They often gather representatives from across the food system, including producers, processors, waste management, urban planners, Extension agents, and nonprofit and for-profit entities with a vested interest in supporting the food system. Remember, everyone has to eat.

While this sounds complicated, sometimes, it can be as simple as ensuring that community gardens are included in a city's strategic plan or providing educational opportunities for citizens so that they know what opportunities lie on their own property. In Missouri, we have something called Cottage Law that allows citizens to sell baked and low-risk foods that have been produced in their own homes. Low-risk means not potentially hazardous to your health if processed improperly. Items such as cheese, meats, salsa, or fermented foods wouldn't be included as an acceptable food to sell under cottage law. Until this law was passed in 2014, there were only sporadic county ordinances that allowed for this. If an ambitious individual wanted to make baked goods, jams, jellies, pastries, or dried herbs to sell directly to consumers, it's perfectly legal to do so up to an income of $50,000. One would still be under the supervision of the local health department, but these opportunities exist for everyone across the state.

Consider also how you're managing your own property. It doesn't matter whether you live in an apartment growing tomatoes in containers or marijuana in the backroom at grandma's house, own a third of an acre or 40 acres, we can all play a part. We all have a responsibility to consider the impact our steward-ship has on our health and the health of our community, as everyone lives down-stream. While using pesticides or inorganic amendments may seem easier and have short-term benefit, supporting and allowing mother nature to balance out the problem should, at least, be considered. A quick Google search goes a long way to appeasing the inquiring mind that wants to manage a plant or food issue more holistically. A great resource for using the right balance in the soil microbi-ome is www.soilfoodweb.com. These folks are quite serious about soil manage-ment and would enjoy the opportunity to help you with yours, and they not only honor the biological approach to food production but also teach it to others.

On the hunger front, a potential solution to the hunger problem is Community Food Utilities (CFU). We have utilities for many of our basic needs: gas, electric, water, and sewer; why not food? Dr. John Ikerd has proposed this understanding as a possible solution to our problem with hunger in America. He believes that hunger is "market failure" that began to occur when we no longer had access to common areas to produce food. People then had to get jobs to pay for food in the grocery store rather than growing their own. While programs like Ozarks Food Harvest are important for our communities, as they have, no doubt, kept many from starving, we still have the overwhelming issue of undernutrition to manage. "If we care enough to eliminate hunger, we must recreate communities of people who accept personal responsibility, to ensure that everyone has access to enough good food," says Ikerd. It can't just be about governmental subsidies. It has to become personal.

The problem now is that it just isn't personal. The COVID-19 crisis was a great example of how the current food system disproportionately affected people with less income. Historically, we had relationships with our neighbors or the butcher down the street, and we relied on each other personally. We had a vested interest in assuring those around us were well fed. One of the early local food groups I worked with was called the Well Fed Neighbor Alliance. It no longer functions under this name but the tag line for their marketing was a bit of genius. "The best defense against hard times is a well-fed neighbor." While multiple meanings can be construed here, it lends credibility to the understanding around the starting of a CFU. Internalizing and personalizing a process around local regenerative food distribution that helps to support its members regardless of income makes a great deal of sense. I suspect that a CFU might also reduce crime rates because of the engagement on the community level. The idea that communities need to rely on federal and state subsidization to feed the hungry needs to be separated from the reality that these programs essentially keep people not only reliant on them but don't necessarily support nutritional status. Finding a community supported alternative needs to become the norm.

These ideas aren't meant to be an all-encompassing list but simply a catalyst for consideration in your own life or community. Many of the examples provided within this section distinctly overlap with more than one other Healthy Food Root/Route. Understanding its significance and applicability is perhaps what's most important rather than which subcategory it falls under. If we begin to nurture behaviors, change our food experiences and food environments, we can facilitate lasting change, not just for us as individuals but for the greater good, making the right choice the easy choice. Continuing to just look at eating healthfully as a performance standard with a possible long-term personal health outcome, we'll inevitably fall short on the opportunities that have been laid before us as connected, social, environmentally concerned citizens.

9.
All Roads Lead Home

Henry Miller, an American author, once said, "A destination is never a place but a new way of seeing things." Our destination needs to be a new way of looking at our health, eating, and the political and environmental influence that food has on this planet before the personal crisis occurs. Most of us get up every day only to do the same thing the same way repeatedly because it's the way we've always done it. Unless something is very wrong, why should we change? What we're doing seems to work pretty well. Maybe it's not perfect but hey, what is? Right? Generally, to decide to do something different, there has to be a significant reason; otherwise, we just keep on doing the same thing. Usually, some sort of event sparks us to ask some questions about how it could be done differently. When it comes to health, it's usually a crisis of some sort, an unexpected diagnosis or hurdle. Deciding to change before the problem exists leaves us healthier, happier, and in a place where we can influence the daily working of our lives.

There's no doubt that food is medicine and can cure, but the wrong food can degrade our health just as quickly. What if we eaters considered changing our belief system or internal narrative around food? What if we realized the magical place that supports our health, the island called Vitality, was already within our reach and all we needed to do was reach out and decide to change a few of our own behaviors, our own direction? No GPS, steering wheel, compass, expensive surgery, or doctor needed.

You see, all health is local. Each of us, with few exceptions, are the product of our immediate environments: home and community. Until the advent of the internet, this was where 99% of our experiences were. We can travel the world wide, but if we come home and flop our bodies on the couch, change nothing about our immediate food environment, and don't have a support network or a vision about our health, circumstances will again dictate what happens to our health repeatedly.

This paradigm shift needs to encourage our society to return to our food roots/routes. In this case, our healthy food roots/routes in order to encourage our overall health to a new, connected, and environmentally conscious place. We need to know how to turn three vining sweet potatoes in our pantry into 10 gallons of sweet potatoes in five months just by cutting them up and placing them in the ground. We need to know how long and at what temperature to ferment kombucha before it turns to vinegar. We need to know what season broccoli grows best in. We need to know what grass-fed beef looks like and why it's an important commodity in the American food system. We need to know how to braid bread because it's fun. Heck, we need to know how to make bread, much less braid it. We need to know how to make bone broth from scratch. We need to know how to save seeds. All these things not only save our food dollars but allow us the opportunity to select purposefully what we eat and keep us in charge of our food, encouraging more confidence in our capabilities in and around our relationship with food. We've become so far removed from our food that it's impacting our health not only from the nutrition perspective but from the connection, community, and environmental perspective as well.

Families and communities that choose to eat together and build lives together, stay together. Tolerance for idiosyncrasies becomes commonplace as we head into the next meal. From the family that chooses to sit down almost every evening, despite what activities are going on, to the every Sunday church or neighborhood gathering building food traditions, staying engaged in activities that center around creating culinary fun in the kitchen, gardening, growing food, and learning create environments that help to keep us connected to our food roots, away from TV computer, and phone screens and engaged in our food environments. This paradigm shift with personal and community decision making needs to occur because we, as individuals, can take charge of this part of our lives, even if state and national policy doesn't support our health. This is a choice that can be made with our food purchasing dollars within our own homes. Our health doesn't have to be a victim of our dysfunctional food system just as our health isn't a victim of our genes.

So, to recap succinctly, the following few changes would have an immediate positive impact on health.

1) Eat meat raised from regenerative farms. If not regenerative, then organic. This reduces the overall amount of antibiotic residues in meats that, in turn, keeps the microbiome less disrupted.

2) Increasing fruit and vegetable consumption with less pesticide residues also helps to keep the microbiome intact and encourages higher phytochemical consumption, which also translates to better health. Again, choose regenerative or organic produce to capitalize on both.

3) Reduce the amount of highly processed foods in the diet. This reduces the possibility of higher total body exposure to foods with limited nutritional value and to some of the chemicals in packaging that can also cause issues with our microbiome and endocrine systems.

4) Choose a water/hydration source that limits the additional exposure to chemicals in groundwater. Consider a filtration system if there are concerns about your local water source.

5) Start cooking as much as possible from scratch at home with real food ingredients defined within these pages.

We Americans are not getting any healthier, and these recommendations will not be found in any dietary guidelines published by any governmental entity.

Many times, we separate the issues that I've brought forward in this book that tie together a healthier person to the healthier planet. The major environmental issues that our planet is challenged by today are directly impacted by our food choices which directly impact our health. If all problems are, in fact, opportunities, this is our opportunity to marry our health with the understanding that even a small personal decision today as one individual can have a huge environmental impact if only 100,000 people decide to do the same thing. That decision can be as simple as buying food from a regenerative farmer or choosing to engage in Healthy Food Roots that support the overall movement toward a healthier you and a healthier planet.

Remember who you are. You're a part of the largest economic engine on the planet. Where will you place your support or spend your money, knowing that it's a vote for your health and that food system?

Call to Action

Think about your current position not only in your own home but also at your job or in the community. Are you a physician? Mother of four? Urban planner? Grocery shopper? Single dad? Bellhop? Or the lawn lady? On the most fundamental level, it doesn't matter. We all need to eat. On the positional level, think about what you could do to facilitate a policy change in your community, work, or home world. My favorite example will always be that of Jason Bauer, the Food Service Director at CoxHealth. He attended the second class of the Cox College internship 13 years ago where he had a healthy indoctrination into the caveats of our food system and how important it is to choose healthy foods. He worked his way up to director of the system, whereby he consistently supported opportunities for local producers until, ultimately, the community relationships were built to support Annabelle's Farm on CoxHealth property. These sorts of projects appear to the community to be an overnight success story but are essentially decades in the making. Jason stood firm on his beliefs and maintained the relationships necessary until the farm came to fruition.

Some of the most sustainable opportunities in local food systems exist because an individual challenged and changed a thought or belief about what was important. Relationships were fostered to support an alliance that built a system rather than individual financial gain. Ultimately, the gains for the community far outweighed the need of the individual, which allowed the system to be supported over time. These are the relationships that need to be forged moving forward with local and regional food systems. These relationships support more than just a single bottom line financial gain. These relationships can be fostered over time to support individual health, local economy, community, as well as the environment, and, ultimately, they don't need to rely on state or federal subsidization to ensure their continued success. Interestingly, this supports the individual in the end, but it's sometimes challenging to see the connections at the outset. Hopefully, the preceded pages helped to pull it together in your minds and hearts.

Perhaps ask yourself, what's your personal and professional sphere of influence? Do you have any influence over food purchasing at home or at work? Do you have any influence over policy making of food purchasing? Do you have any influence on what gets planted in landscaping at home or work? Do you have any influence on community planning around community or food endeavors? What are you willing to influence in an effort to preserve not only your own health, but the health of your family and the community around you? This could mean reaching out to local producers to support a supply chain that brings local grass-fed beef hamburgers in the cafeteria, supporting a local producer's farmers' market on premise for employees to enjoy, or perhaps sourcing local, hydroponic lettuce for the salad bar. Help plant an herb garden at your place of work to inspire folks to eat more herbs. The list of influential possibilities is, in fact, endless. And every small change counts.

When we realize the damage that has been done to our planet, health, and communities all in the name of producing more food that, many times, doesn't even make it to the mouth of an individual, we should seriously question our next steps. What can we each do as an individual that provides a sense of purpose through eating? The act of eating, whether we like it or not, has, in fact, become more than a nourishing act; it's political. Where our food dollars go, so goes the support for tomorrow's food supply. What would you like your food dollars to support? Our society of convenience needs to replace the mindset that it's quickest and easiest to go to the drive thru with the understanding that this act continues support for the industrialized food system. The paradigm has to shift toward regenerative, food centricity, slowing our lives down, and planning ahead.

Large Steps Forward

The biggest, most cost-prohibitive problem with our food system is, by far, the loss of family-owned farmland. Our farmland has become vulnerable to development due to the expansion of our cities. Large multinational corporations are buying up farmland close to these cities, offering generational farms large sums of money as property values increase, making it more appealing to sell rather than keep the family farm in operation. Farms are no longer being passed from generation to generation as upcoming generations no longer see a life on the farm, or the life they see involves long hours and heartbreak, giving in to the pressure of financial gain over tradition. Remember the example from Washington County, ME. This is why there was a 16% reduction in farmland from 2012 to 2017 in that county. If one were to pull farmland statistics in rural counties, it's the same story all over America.

The good news is that this issue is being recognized by some major organizations that want to make a difference. Some of the more promising programs include those that protect our farmland from becoming a part of the urban sprawl. Programs that buy, protect and sell farmland that keep the land not only as farm over the long term but also support sustainable or regenerative agriculture ensures that this land will, at least, not become part of the growing problem of improperly managed soil and/or be sold for further development and a permanent installment of pavement that contributes to runoff. Local policy efforts and farmland protection are a joint effort between local governments and nongovernmental entities working together to stave off future developments that move our society away from farm life and tradition. If this concern speaks to you, and you have farmland that you would like to keep in farming, consider reaching out to one of the following organizations that have programs to keep family farmland in production, some specific to regenerative or sustainable agriculture protection.

https://www.onestl.org/toolkit/list/practice/farmland-preservation East-West Council of Governments

https://farmland.org/ American Farmland Trust

https://www.conservationfund.org/our-work/cities/farmland-protection The Conservation Fund

This is, by no means, an extensive list. Please check around you to access all resources available. And if located in the James River Basin in SW Missouri, consider reaching out to the Watershed Committee of the Ozarks to see what might be worked in cooperation with their new funding.

We've also taken large steps forward with the organic regenerative farming standard. While the organic standard itself has become somewhat compromised through a systemic relaxing of the rules, I didn't go into any detail in this book purposefully. This could be an entire book by itself. The regenerative standard still has no official definition from our federal government. Just like anything, this lack of standard leaves it open to interpretation, which can be either a good or a bad thing, depending upon who decides to assign the terminology of the "regenerative" farming practice. Basically, anyone can call what they do regenerative. Our job is essentially to protect not the standard per se but the agricultural understanding of what regenerative actually means. I believe however that what really matters is how it was defined in Chapter 3 in the Regenerative Ecosystems section. If we focus on the soil, regeneration of the soil, nurturing the microbiome of the soil rather than degrading the soil, the rest will fall into place. When we, as consumers, become aware of what regenerative actually means as well as recognizing what its influence is, growing a more nutrient-dense and delicious food item, reducing CO_2 in the atmosphere, and keeping our waterways pristine, there's no downside to supporting this. None. Conversely, there's a great purpose behind this. Eating to save the planet and our health.

Farm Bill 2023

While the relationships we nurture on a community level that support the concept of the WIN/WIN/WIN mutuality toward local and regional food systems over time are perhaps the best option, what if there were substantial funding to support this instead of an industrialized system? If we grow and eat what we subsidize in this country, the next Farm Bill coming due in 2023 has an opportunity to support not only the family farm but also the worker as well as the environment. This, in turn, supports the health of our people on the multiple levels discussed in the pages of this book. If the current subsidies were gradually shifted towards programs that keep the family-run regenerative farm intact with direct support for local and regional food systems, our access to real food has the potential to change dramatically. More specifically, the 2023 Farm Bill could:

1. Support conceptualization and infrastructure around Community Food Utility development within individual communities that show interest in approaching the issue of food insecurity quite differently than just providing food to the less fortunate. Allow communities to define this for themselves. It has to be accomplished on this level.

2. Support small, diversified farms both financially as well as providing additional insurance options for them so they can expand their markets.

3. Support local and regional food system infrastructure with a particular focus on processing of proteins or meat products, and additional financial support for agrihoods and food hubs.

4. Provide additional funding for food hubs that provide regenerative food as a source for SNAP and WIC programs. This could work in cooperation with numbers 1 and 3. Ensure that those who breach antitrust laws will be actively sued, prosecuted, and fined within a timeframe that benefits those who suffer the most when this occurs: the farmer in competitive markets.

5. Support programs that keep century farms in regenerative agricultural production like Buy, Protect, Sell.

The current Farm Bill has massive subsidies toward keeping the current system in place. While dismantling the current system abruptly would likely have far reaching and unpredictably devastating effects, the gentle nudge toward a system that supports regeneration of our land could do nothing but support real food production. If even 25% of the Farm Bill went toward regenerative agriculture and supporting local and regional food systems, this would represent slightly over $216 billion or close to $214 billion more than is currently being shunted to this system. Is this too much to ask in the land of plenty and a capitalistic system that supports the rich getting richer?

Make Food Personal

If one wants to succeed in improving health, it has to be personal. Our lives must be made food centric or food centered with "conscious eating" and decision making around maintaining a relationship with our food rather than allowing it to become an afterthought. When I think back to my childhood, I realize that I was pretty fortunate to have a family that ate reasonably well. Our family started connecting to our food through gardening and canning. My father, to this day, at 82 years of age still has a garden with greens and herbs. Much of the time, when our family gets together, it's spent planning, cooking, and eating. As I write this, I know when they read this, it will strike them odd that that's what we do.

My subconscious internal food narrative has always been that food should be fun, well thought out, and good for me. This doesn't mean that I eat perfectly every single day. As a food professional, I'm not even sure what that means. I drank my fair share of diet Pepsi and ate microwave popcorn back in the day, even lazing through label reading with new food products on the market enamored by the fun packaging and empty marketing illusions. I used to promote soy products and canola oil in my consultations until I found out about the environmental impacts of these crops as well as the potential negative health outcomes hidden by the misinformation put out by the industry.

What it does mean though, is that a component of every day involves voluntary planning around how to stay healthy with access to real food that nourishes my body rather than degrading my health. Armed with the knowledge and understanding that food is more than just something that nourishes the body, it makes those extra steps to head to the farmers' market or grow some food of my own that much more meaningful. Walking forward with the peace of mind that my food choices are also helping to keep the planet healthy as well as support the community and a local food economy isn't a small deal!

What's your internal food narrative? Does it match up with the choices that you make every day? Find your sweet spot for real food in your life right now. While a little bit of competition is healthy, it doesn't matter if it totally aligns with what your neighbor or friends do. Everyone has a limit to what they can take on at any given time. Do what you can. Find your once-a-week go-to recipes, the crutch that you can lean on when things get stressful. Life will always find a way to provide opportunities for excuses for choosing an unhealthier path. Don't give it a foothold in your food journey.

It took me 20 years and tons of research to start paying attention to my own health in an additionally beneficial way. I finally found myself taking the extra steps and preparation to ensure that I had a successful food day. This sometimes meant prepping food the night before, eating leftovers so I didn't have to be concerned with food tomorrow, or just having a game plan in my head for the coming day. For me, this also meant feeling better, so it became an easier choice the better I felt. It took time to weed through what worked well for me and with the understanding that the same therapeutic interventions don't work for everyone. There are some good basic places to start like with the Mediterranean diet and clean eating with real, regeneratively raised food, but, again, one size doesn't fit all, so please keep that in mind when meandering toward your next food adventure. It takes consistency over time to make a difference in our health.

So, ask yourself, what's the next step for improving your health? What's your food journey? Whatever you decide, instead of engaging in the hundreds of reasons why you can't do something, just start doing it. Choose a Food Root/

Route and start walking forward. Most everyone has access to the internet. Start researching your next step and implement one action around your plan. Food should be fun and engaging, and when it is, the decision to make those extra efforts becomes quite simple. This helps to make the right choice, the easy choice. Find a way to engage with your food that keeps you wanting to go back and fine tune some more. Once you get started, you might find even more ideas that haven't been mentioned in this book. Everyone is in a different place in their food journey. Find someone to hold you accountable for your decisions who understands what you're trying to accomplish and helps to provide a sense of shared purpose. Don't be afraid to fail, as, at least, you got started and know what doesn't work for you. Share your successes and failures but most of all, love your food journey.